Keats's Anatomy of Melancholy

Keat's Anatomy of Melancholy

*Lamia, Isabella, The Eve of St Agnes,
And Other Poems* (1820)

R. S. White

EDINBURGH
University Press

Edinburgh University Press is one of the leading university presses in the UK. We publish academic books and journals in our selected subject areas across the humanities and social sciences, combining cutting-edge scholarship with high editorial and production values to produce academic works of lasting importance. For more information visit our website: edinburghuniversitypress.com

Edinburgh University Press Ltd
The Tun – Holyrood Road
12(2f) Jackson's Entry
Edinburgh EH8 8PJ

First published in hardback by Edinburgh University Press 2020

Typeset in 10.5/13 Adobe Sabon by
Servis Filmsetting Ltd, Stockport, Cheshire,
and printed and bound by CPI Group (UK) Ltd,
Croydon, CR0 4YY

A CIP record for this book is available from the British Library

ISBN 978 1 4744 8045 1 (hardback)
ISBN 978 1 4744 8046 8 (paperback)
ISBN 978 1 4744 8047 5 (webready PDF)
ISBN 978 1 4744 8048 2 (epub)

Contents

List of Illustrations

Acknowledgements

I am especially grateful to Nicholas Roe, John Barnard and Beth Lau for their abundance of scholarly generosity in reading portions of the book and offering valuable insights, suggestions and corrections. I am also penitent to have presumed so much on their time and attention, my only excuse being that reader response critics crave responses from readers. Needless to say, all remaining errors and infelicities are my own alone. Thanks to John Goodridge for unflagging moral support and sharing ideas from his well of knowledge of Keats and John Clare, and for his critical acumen, and humane wisdom. I owe a large debt to Ken Page and Frankie Kubicki who allowed me to spend many hours over some years poring over Keats's copy of Burton in the inspiring setting of the Keats-Shelley Memorial House in Hampstead. Gareth Evans, formerly of the Chelsea Botanic Garden where Keats studied plants, and whose website on 'botanical and cultural histories' is rich with information and insights, freely shared his unrivalled knowledge of medical botany in Keats's time. Others offered specific information, help, or all-important encouragement, most of whom have no doubt long forgotten their contributions. These include in particular Giuseppe Albano, Catherine Belsey, Martin Dodsworth, Hrileena Ghosh, Claire Lamont, Michael Levine, Lo Ka Tat, Jon Mee, Meiko O'Halloran, Li Ou, Ciara Rawnsley, Erin Sullivan, Maurice Whelan, the late Robert Woof, and many others including former students at Newcastle upon Tyne and Western Australia, from whom I have learned much about the unexpected individuality of a range of 'reader responses' in practice. My association with the Australian Research Council Centre of Excellence for the History of Emotions (2011–2018) provided congenial company and valuable interdisciplinary discussions, in particular with Louis Charland and Jennifer Radden. The Australian Research Council also funded two years' research leave to research the book. Much of the final stretch of writing came with the uniquely gratifying opportunity offered by election to the Magdalen College for Senior Visiting Research Fellow in 2018, allowing me to inhabit old haunts in the Bodleian, Radcliffe Camera and English Faculty Library, and enabled me at last to meet Laurie Maguire whose work I have long admired. Over the years, through the much appreciated efforts of Mark Howe, I have also enjoyed annual migratory accommodation in another old haunt, Holywell Manor, Balliol College, which always brings back happy memories. Over a period of years, the resources of the British Library, the Wellcome Library, and the Reid Library at the University of Western Australia have been invaluable. I am grateful to the Houghton Library at Harvard University, the British Library, the Wellcome Library, the New York Public Libraries, and the Art Gallery of South Australia (one of my favourite places in undergraduate days) for permissions to reproduce images. In writing on 'Isabella', I have unavoidably drawn (in revised form) on material which I published in 'Keats, Mourning and Melancholia', *John Keats and the Medical Imagination*, edited by Nicholas Roe (London: Palgrave, 2017), 129–52, and I am grateful for the editor's permission to do so. Quotations from Keats's 1820 volume are taken from the facsimile of this text, while his other poems are quoted from John Barnard's Penguin edition, another constant companion since undergraduate days, sundry copies replaced as each one disintegrated through constant over-reading. Finally, I am grateful to the Edinburgh University Press, their very efficient and congenial publishing team and the two generous anonymous readers, for making it possible to publish the book in the bicentenary year of Keats's precious volume.

Unity

To E. B. from J. K.

LAMIA,

ISABELLA,

THE EVE OF ST. AGNES,

AND

OTHER POEMS.

———

BY JOHN KEATS,

AUTHOR OF ENDYMION.

———

LONDON:

PRINTED FOR TAYLOR AND HESSEY,

FLEET-STREET.

1820.

1.1 Title page of the copy inscribed to Fanny Brawne from John Keats, Houghton Library at Harvard University, citation number Keats *EC8.K2262.820 l(F).

Chapter 1

Lamia, Isabella, The Eve of St Agnes, And Other Poems (1820) as a Unified Volume

The historic significance of Keats's volume of poems published in 1820 under the title *Lamia, Isabella, The Eve of St Agnes, And Other Poems* is hardly in doubt. Walter Jackson Bate in 1963 described the collection as 'in many ways perhaps the most remarkable single volume to be published by any poet during the past century and a half, if we leave aside collected works published by poets in their old age . . .'.[1] However, Bate's biographical interest lay not in following up this insight but in tracing the chronology of Keats's poetic development poem-by-poem in the light of his life story. More recently, Kelvin Everest in the entry on Keats in the *Oxford Dictionary of National Biography* has written, 'This collection is now recognised as among the most important works of English poetry ever published'. Yet it has still only rarely been analysed in these terms as a single collection, and although 'The Eve of St. Agnes' and the odes are justly famous and well-loved, they are usually encountered by readers as individual poems in anthologies. In most editions of Keats's poetry, they are divorced from the context of the collection as a whole and presented chronologically in a progress from 'juvenilia' to triumphant 'maturity'. In the case of this, Keats's second collection, it may paradoxically be the memorable brilliance of individual poems which has distracted attention from their inclusion in a single-authored anthology, despite the fact that this consideration provides facets of subtle interrelatedness between the poems which reveal new meanings. Recontextualised by keeping company with each other, rubbing shoulders with poems other than just the universally celebrated ones, and arranged by author and publishers in a considered order, the whole is greater than the parts. The one important qualification whose importance I shall argue for, is that evidence suggests that Keats intended 'Ode on Melancholy' to be the final poem in the collection, and that the inclusion of 'Hyperion. A Fragment' was a publisher's decision which he resisted. This, I suggest, makes a very significant difference to the structure intended by Keats. In other words, Keats's collection in a sense has never been presented as he wished.

An important thread, which I intend to follow through the volume as at least one of its major thematic concerns, is the persistent emphasis on different shades and types of melancholy, an ancient, major medical condition and changing literary preoccupation in Renaissance and Romantic poetry. This affective condition was considerably richer and more complex before and during Keats's time than is suggested by today's paler meaning of the word 'melancholy'. As a dominant passion in the Renaissance, it could include a spectrum of emotions ranging from suicidal despair to manic hilarity, and many in between, including artistic exhilaration, different kinds of love, and excessive religious enthusiasm. In this design, the clinching closure to the 1820 volume comes with 'Ode on Melancholy', which attributes value to the emotional state and embraces it as a form of creative inspiration. The theme of melancholy, as I hope to show, reached Keats from different cultural perspectives offered by his life circumstances and temperament, his medical training, and his reading of literature, including eighteenth century graveyard poetry and Gothic novels. More specifically, during 1819 when Keats wrote and collected the bulk of poems in *1820*, he was also enthusiastically reading Robert Burton's *The Anatomy of Melancholy*, a quirky, encyclopaedic and gigantic study, which was written as a Renaissance contribution to medical knowledge but had been revitalised by Romantic literary figures. Viewed in this way, Keats's 1820 volume stands as a celebration and personal analysis of a major, longstanding Western cultural and medical tradition which was close to the poet's heart. It is his own, brief 'anatomy of melancholy'. Keats spoke of the artist's stance as one that 'does no harm from its relish of the dark side of things',[2] and this volume demonstrates his contemplative, 'camelion' ambivalences, turning subjects this way and that to inspect their dark and light sides, melancholy and joy, states which are by turns contrasted, explored, and synthesised.

One impediment to considering the context and framework of the whole volume that Keats envisaged, as pointed out recently by Grant Scott,[3] has been the modern critical 'tyranny' to value above all the 'sacred unity of the odes', to the neglect of the other poems.[4] It is an emphasis which Keats himself may not have anticipated. Edmund Blunden may have been the most influential in transmitting the preeminence of the odes, since his (admittedly brief) *Writers and their Works* study of Keats mentions only the odes from the 1820 volume.[5] Midcentury critical works by Earl Wasserman and Helen Vendler[6] in particular, consolidated the emergence of a modern canon of 'Keats's

Major Poems' giving prime consideration to the odes, in particular 'Ode to a Nightingale', 'Ode on a Grecian Urn' and 'To Autumn', and (in Wasserman's case) 'The Eve of St Agnes' and 'Lamia', though even the latter has slipped down in critical estimation. The other poems in the 1820 volume were silently relegated to a rank less than 'major'.

Changes in taste have meant that romance *epyllia* such as 'Lamia' and 'Isabella' have long since fallen out of fashion, despite their celebrity in Romantic times, although 'The Eve of St. Agnes' has fared better. They were in vogue particularly in the circle of Leigh Hunt, John Hamilton Reynolds, 'Barry Cornwall' (Bryan Procter), and Robert Merry's Della Cruscan group, but the fashion did not last long. It is significant that in the title to his book Keats highlighted the longer poems, indicating that his ordering is at least partially based on genre. Romantic narratives are followed by *Other Poems* including odes and *rondeaux*, and if we include the 'Hyperion' fragment, a portion of an epic. Perhaps the order indicates an intention to foreground the longer poems as a potential selling point with a particular audience in mind. The modern emphasis on the odes would not necessarily have occurred to Keats himself, and it may distract and mislead us when considering his collection as a whole. It is noteworthy that self-evident supremacy of the odes seems not to have been the verdict of either Keats himself or his contemporary readers, since reviewers at the time, whether sympathetic or critical, do not prioritise them. Attention was focused mainly on the three romances in the title, and on the 'Hyperion' fragment, which contemporaries, including Shelley and Byron, singled out for admiration but regarded as different from the other poems in the volume.[7] If they had been able to read the later, completely revised fragment, which was not published until long after Keats's death in 1848 under the name *The Fall of Hyperion. A Dream*, they would have found their impression justified, that the fragmentary draft points towards a future, different and compelling epic in its own right, which was also never brought to completion by Keats. Although the inclusion of 'Hyperion. A Fragment' may have compromised the integrity of the collection as Keats envisaged it, yet in some ways, especially in the depiction of the Titans' despondent state, it can be seen as consistent with the volume's overall spirit of melancholy, which in itself is not surprising, since Keats was working on it on-and-off before and during the same period as he was putting together the collection and reading Burton.

In addition to the problems of interpretation raised by the later celebrity given to the odes, and by the inclusion of the fragment, many modern editions tend to obscure the unity of the volume further by rarely republishing *1820* as a volume in its own right. Instead, it is much more common to find the individual poems presented according to dates of composition, which is not the order adopted in *1820*. There has been one photographically reproduced facsimile reprint without annotations, now held in the Bodleian Library (shelfmark Don.f.100), of *Lamia, Isabella, The Eve of St Agnes, And Other Poems*, which is used for quotations here.[8] The volume was also reproduced, again without annotations, explanations, or even an Introduction, in a short-lived 'Penguin First Editions' series, which included anthologies by Rupert Brooke, Robert Burns, A. E. Houseman, D. H. Lawrence, Wordsworth and Coleridge, and W. B. Yeats.[9] Apart from these, only one (very lightly) annotated single volume text of *1820* was published, as long ago as 1909.[10] Meanwhile, the major, standard annotated editions of the 'complete poems', such as those by Douglas Bush, Miriam Allott, John Barnard (in his earlier Penguin edition), and Jack Stillinger, reprint the poems in order of presumed composition rather than retaining the order of the 1820 volume, a practice which places the emphasis on Keats's development as a poet rather than on the collection. There are exceptions in some 'complete works', such as John Barnard's most recent 'Oxford Twenty-first Century' edition, Jeffrey N. Cox's 'Norton Critical' edition, and Edward Hirsch's Random House edition, which at least preserve the order of poems in the anthology. But again, the footnotes and annotations emphasise the dates of composition, and there is little sustained analysis of the poet's chosen organisation of his collection. Jack Stillinger was certainly aware of the 'volume' approach since, as we shall shortly see, he was keenly aware that the poems in Keats's first collection in 1817 had been thematically connected and arranged, and he also offers pithy comments on the ordering of *1820*. But in his role as editor, he once again chose the model of presenting the individual poems in chronological order. Meanwhile, Keats's major biographers, Walter Jackson Bate, Robert Gittings, and Nicholas Roe understandably also focus mainly on the poet's development. Gittings devoted his book *John Keats: The Living Year* to the composition of the individual poems, most of them written during 1819, but considering them individually and out of the context of the 1820 volume.[11] This may seem to both editors and biographers an obvious and illuminating strategy, but, I argue, is interpretatively incomplete, since the poems can be reinterpreted in the light of their selection and placement in the volume.

There is a wealth of evidence, both biographical and intrinsic to the volume, suggesting that Keats took pains to place these apparently 'occasional' poems into a sequence which is interconnected stylistically and thematically, and it was not his design to present simply his 'best poems' in either random or chronological order. This has consequences for a reader in interpreting the volume as a whole and as it stands. Each poem is illuminated by the others in turn, and by the overarching existence of the volume as a whole. Moreover, the common editorial methodology overshadows other open questions. Why, for example, does the volume include earlier poems that were not part of the undisputed flowering of Keats's poetry in 1819, works such as 'Isabella' (Keats had reservations about its quality), 'Lines on the Mermaid Tavern' and 'Robin Hood' both written early in 1818 as epistolary jokes in correspondence with Reynolds? And why did Keats not include 'La Belle Dame Sans Merci', while at one stage seriously weighing up including the very lightweight 'Song of Four Faeries'? It would seem that the contents and their ordering in the book have significance and raise questions beyond the biographical.

As in editions and biographies, so in critical studies, the unity of *1820* is rarely considered. However, on the general question of a poetic collection having an internal coherence which surpasses the individual poems, I take encouragement from two brief but suggestive precedents. Stillinger, in his chapter 'The Order of Poems in Keats's First Volume' in *The Hoodwinking of Madeline and Other Essays on Keats's Poems*, argues for a planned, thematic integrity in Keats's earliest volume, *Poems* (1817):

> While it should not surprise anyone that poets do frequently give serious thought to the arrangement of their poems, the fact is that we almost never consider either their intentions or the effects critically ... [critics] seldom suggest why Keats printed one poem before or after another. The readiest explanation for this neglect is that biographers and biographically oriented critics, naturally unwilling to discuss the poems twice – at both composition and publication – have almost universally chosen to treat the poems chronologically according to composition.[12]

He suggests that Keats's preoccupation in *Poems* (1817) was with 'poetry itself, with a centring on the question of whether he can and should be a poet'.[13] *1820* is, however, altogether darker, focusing on confronting emotional adversities, loss, and consolation. Stillinger did not go on in any detail to apply his logic to the infinitely richer 1820 volume, perhaps sensing the job would be considerably larger and more complex than for the 1817 one. But he does offer some suggestive *obiter dicta* about the order in which Keats chose to present the poems in *1820*, especially the odes: 'And whatever the explanation, it is surely no accident that *Ode to a Nightingale* and *Ode on a Grecian Urn* were printed before instead of (as they seem to have been written) after *Ode to Psyche*, in the same volume' (p. 2). Stillinger's overall interpretation of the volume mirrors his reading of Keats's poetic development as a whole: 'Arranged as they are, the poems show a progressive abandonment of the ideal and accept-ance of the natural world, and a gradual movement from irresolution to resolution' (p. 116); from Lycius's involvement in 'an illusory ideal' through to 'the two final odes, 'To Autumn' and 'Melancholy', with their focus on the natural world and unequivocal acceptance of it' (pp. 116–17). Meanwhile, Neil Fraistat in a fine chapter of his book, *The Poem and the Book*, suggests that the 1820 collection shows 'sophis-ticated organization' and that the 'poems are positioned without refer-ence to their chronological order of composition'.[14] This he argues by comparing a number of poetic collections published between 1790 and 1830, showing that such systematisation is not at all uncommon in Keats's period. His chapter-length study of Keats's *1820* finds stylistic links between the poems, in arguing for a complex, detailed ordering in *1820*:

> as the reader moves sequentially from the opening "Lamia" to the conclud-ing "Hyperion," he discovers a complex system of verbal echoes, transi-tional links, and thematic progressions through which each poem revises the meaning of its predecessor.[15]

Fraistat goes on to examine each poem in order, tracing 'verbal echoes, transitional links, and thematic progressions'. The dominant theme, he proposes, is a repeated sequence of enchantment and disenchantment in each poem. I am grateful to have Fraistat's pioneering chapter to build upon, but hope to foreground another theme, melancholy, which I believe is just as prominent and has many subtle consequences for the collection as a whole and the ordering of the poems in it. That Fraistat and Stillinger were 'on the same page' in their approaches to poetic col-lections was shown when Stillinger reviewed Fraistat's book favourably, arguing again that,

> The constructing of books of poems, involving choices of contents, arrange-ment, and format, is a topic that has occupied poets and publishers a great deal but scholars hardly at all. In traditional study of the English Romantics we routinely place poems in such biographical, historical, and literary con-texts as the life of the author, the chronology of the author's work, the whole body of the author, the traditions and genres and conventions of the time (and earlier and later), and so on and on. Only rarely do we consider what might be thought the most obvious context of all, the original collections in which the poems were presented to the public.[16]

This remains broadly true today regarding Keats's 1820 collection.

The Significance of Poetic Collections

Fraistat has separately compiled a set of scholarly essays on significant anthologies by mainly non-Romantic authors from Virgil and Ovid to Sylvia Plath.[17] Michael Gamer has followed up in his recent book on the phenomenon of the Romantic 're-collection', which he defines as 'the authorized, transformational reprinting of works that have appeared earlier in some form' for commercial purposes. Gamer does not include Keats's *1820* in his analysis since it is not a 're-collection' in the strict sense because, with the exceptions of 'Ode to a Nightingale' and 'Ode on a Grecian Urn', the poems had not already been published. However, similar general points can be made about Keats's activity in putting together the 1820 volume:

> Sometimes adding new material to previously published works and sometimes not, a re-collection is never merely a new edition of an older book. Rather, it gathers its component parts and presents them in new ways, transforming the assembled contents – through combination and juxtaposition, revision and re-ordering, repricing and repackaging – so as effectively to produce a new work . . . [offering] a chance to produce a more capacious account of literary production and reception by shifting our critical gaze from initial composition to what comes after.[18]

Gamer coins the phrase 'self-canonization' to describe what the author is attempting in anthologising his or her work. His phrase might perhaps complement Stephen Greenblatt's notion of 'self-fashioning' in the Renaissance, a literary equivalent of how an author wishes to be read and remembered.[19] The distinctive genre of a poetic collection is, in Gamer's words, the author's attempt to provide 'at once a calculated publishing venture and a constitutive monument in progress'.[20] In Keats's case, *1820* was intended as a step towards his own ambitious aspiration: 'I think I shall be among the English Poets after my death'.[21] His statement bears at least two senses, that his volume will sit on bookshelves beside those of Spenser, Shakespeare and Milton, and that his poems will in turn be anthologised in such popular series as John Bell's *Poets of Great Britain* (1776–82).[22] A chapter in Gamer's *Romanticism and Self-Canonization* demonstrates how numerous and popular were such anthologies from the 1770s onwards, citing Keats's hope as 'arguably the most suggestive statement regarding standard collections'.[23] But first, Keats realised, he needed to produce an anthology of his own works as a step towards fulfilling his prophecy, necessarily aiming at the judgment of posterity since such collections, by convention, did not include living poets. At the least, the 1820 volume was surely conceived as one 'constitutive monument' towards his longer goal, which was certainly reached 'after [his] death'.

There are a handful of single-authored collections whose status as unified entities has been widely accepted as surpassing in significance the individual works they contain within their covers. In these, the effect of the whole is acknowledged to be greater than, and different from, the constituent poems. Historically, publication of such a volume is identified in retrospect as an 'event' in the history of the book. Among these we might include sonnet sequences tracing a love affair, such as Dante's *La Vita Nuova* (1294), Sidney's *Astrophel to Stella* (1580s), and Spenser's *Amoretti* (1595) which traces the events of a single year of 365 days, and series of interconnected quasi-narrative 'tales' such as Chaucer's *The Canterbury Tales* (1380s) and Crabbe's *The Village* (1783) and *The Borough* (1810), building up a social environment through various characters. George Herbert's *The Temple* (1633) provides the clearest example of a structure based on a specific concept completely divorced from the (unknown) order of composition, following as it does the sequence of Christian rituals during the year: Advent, Nativity, Ash Wednesday, Lent, Holy Week, Easter, Ascension, Whitsun and others.[24] Other 'landmark', iconic collections are recognisably based on different principles of selection and ordering such as themes or concepts, amongst them Charlotte Smith's *Elegiac Sonnets* (1783), Burns's *Poems, Chiefly in the Scottish Dialect* (1786), Wordsworth and Coleridge's *Lyrical Ballads* (1798, and 're-collected' in 1800[25]), Yeats's *Responsibilities* (1914) and *The Tower* (1928), T. S. Eliot's *The Waste Land and Other Poems* (1922), and Plath's *Ariel* (1965). In each case the significant 'occasion' is the publication of the collection, surpassing and superseding the sequence of 'mini-occasions' on which the poems were written, usually (so far as we know) in a different order from the one presented in the collection. Fraistat has explained further:

> the book – with all of its informing contexts – is the meeting ground for poet and reader, the 'situation' in which its constituent texts occur. As such, the book is constantly conditioning the reader's responses, activating various sets of what semioticians call 'interpretive codes' A fundamental assumption of such an approach is that the decisions poets make about the presentation of their works play a meaningful role in the poetic process and, hence, ought to figure in the reading process. Studied within the context of their original volumes, poems reveal a fuller textuality, which is to say, an *inter*textuality.[26]

In the same book, Earl Miner uses the term 'integrated collections' to describe such volumes.[27] Milton's *Poems* (1645), which contains his sonnets and other shorter works, including *Comus* and *Lycidas*, presents a different variation. The poems were written over a twenty-year period, and Milton changed the order of sonnets in his three editions of the volume, offering proof that he was consciously thinking about the issue of internal development in the volume.[28] This was routinely the practice also of Wordsworth who, in Stephen Gill's words, 'altered the presentation of his poems from edition to edition'.[29] The most famous case of a poetic collection is also the most intriguing. A whole scholarly industry has been built on the question whether or not Shakespeare planned, executed, and authorised his *Sonnets Never Before Imprinted* (1609) as a unified volume, a genuine narrative sequence, randomly selected, or by the publisher and not the author.

Critical works have been devoted exclusively to such volumes as a whole. Dylan Thomas's pithy 'Note', prefacing his volume *Collected Poems*, suggests one principle of selection, based only on quality: 'This book contains most of the poems I have written, and all, up to the present year [1952], that I wish to preserve'. The order does not seem to matter so much as the presumed excellence of each poem. D. H. Lawrence made different authorial decisions, as he explains in his own 'Note' in 1928.[30] *Rhyming Poems* and *Unrhyming Poems* suggest selection on grounds of form, while other volumes comprise 'sequences' on certain subjects, such as *Birds, Beasts and Flowers*, and *Pansies*. Lawrence's *Last Poems* indicates a biographical principle, while *Uncollected Poems* suggests the simple criterion is that these ones have not previously been included in a collection. There are, then, many different principles of selection but in his 'Note' Lawrence justifies also a chronological ordering in each 'collection' to 'make up a biography of an emotional and inner life' of the author. This in turn illuminates Lawrence's view of the relation between his life and his creativity, since his usual practice was to develop in either poetic or novel form his thought processes as a spontaneous recording of a 'soul biography', until the particular vein of writing was exhausted, or until he turned to another subject, style or theme. This philosophy appears not to be the case in Keats's 1820 volume, since its ordering is not chronological.

Looking beyond collections made by individual poets, there are 'landmark' volumes of poems by sundry writers, selected by an editor who adopts a curatorial role, whose preferences and taste provide the main principle of selection, as in an art exhibition. *Golden Treasury of English Songs and Lyrics* collected by Francis Turner Palgrave, known universally as 'Palgrave's Golden Treasury' (1861–91), is an example. Looking beyond poetry, there are prose collections of short stories, where again the significance of the whole is regarded as greater than its component parts, for example, Edgar Alan Poe's *Tales of the Grotesque and Arabesque* (1840). In his Preface Poe proposes as his 'thesis', 'terror of the soul'. Collections by Guy de Maupassant such as *Contes du jours et de la nuit* (1885) and James Joyce's *Dubliners* (1914), announce in their very titles thematic concentration and principles of selection inviting guided readings. All these examples raise their own questions about why the contents are presented in a certain order, and by asking such questions and providing a range of answers, scholarship has opened up a variety of potential readings which enhance our understanding. The main point is that they are accepted as autonomous and significant publishing 'events'. The courtesy has not yet been extended to Keats's *Lamia, Isabella, The Eve of St Agnes, And Other Poems* (1820), which belongs in this distinguished company of historically important anthologies, even while the immense influence of its individual poems has commanded sustained critical analysis.

The importance of context for literary interpretation might be illustrated by considering 'Ode to a Nightingale'. Charles Brown's story of its apparently automatic composition under the plum tree in the Wentworth Place garden is a colourful and perhaps apocryphal tale, destined to illustrate romantic inspiration in spontaneous composition. Relying on a twenty-year old memory, Brown recounts how Keats entered the house from a morning spent under the plum tree in the garden with 'scraps of paper in his hand, and these he was quietly thrusting behind the books', revealing them only one by one with apparent reluctance.[31] When read with this scenario in mind, the ode acquires a part of its meaning from the myth, created from an anecdotal biographical revelation of the post-compositional diffidence of a genius unaware of the importance of his poem. The story has been doubted by textual scholars, but persists in colouring readings of the poem. Another historical context is Joseph Severn's famous painting, *Keats Listening to a Nightingale on Hampstead Heath*. Created in about 1845, over twenty-five years after the event, this adds different nuances to readings of the poem. Here the poet sits rapt and transported, eyes gazing upwards, an open notebook at his side. Crucially, Severn removes Keats from Brown's domestic morning setting, and places him instead in the windswept landscape of Hampstead Heath against a sky of dramatically scudding clouds, while a full moon peering through the branches denotes twilight. The poet is memorably placed in a wilder version of romantic nature than Brown's homely description evokes, creating quite different associations. Closer to the time (1823–5), Severn had painted Keats reading in the drawing room, recalling that occasion in ways that add yet another layer of context:

> This was at the time he first felt ill & had written the Ode to a Nightingale ^1819^ on the morn[ing] of my visit to Hampstead – I found him sitting

with the two chairs as I have painted him & I was struck with the first real symptom[s] of sadness in Keats so finely expressed in that Poem. —[32]

An emotional state, 'symptoms of sadness' and awareness of illness, add more projected meanings on the poem. It must be added that Severn was writing even longer after the event than Brown, in an 1859 letter (22 December) to George Scharf, founder of the National Portrait Gallery, indicating that hindsight is another interpretive frame.

Keats published the ode some months later in *The Annals of Fine Art* (July, 1819), which suggests that he himself at this stage placed it in a context that adds a different range of potential meanings altogether. This context suggests that it should be read not primarily as a 'nature poem' nor as wholly emotionally expressive, but that its primary subject is art. Finally, Keats placed it in *1820*, where it acquires yet more reflected associations from the company it keeps, and by the light it sheds itself on the adjacent and surrounding poems, as we shall see in Chapter 6. The 'Ode' is also replete with allusions to other writers, mainly Shakespeare, and if these are noticed, yet more layers of intertextuality and contexts are revealed. As in the case of repeated performances of *Hamlet*, can we confidently claim 'Ode to a Nightingale' is the 'same work' on each reading or performance, irrespective of context? In interpreting the volume, it is necessary to draw upon different areas of scholarly expertise, those of biographer, textual scholar, literary historian, and literary critic, in dealing with an apparently 'static' text, yet one that 'moves' in response to varying perspectives, through time, occasions, conscious ordering, and new critical readings.

When dealing with works such as those by Shakespeare and Keats there are no single or final interpretations. Analysis must shift according to changing perspectives, cultural and literary contexts. David Harlan, intellectual historian, describes such works as 'indeterminate', 'multidimensional, omni-significant, inexhaustible, perpetually new . . .'.[33] More recently and speaking of Shakespeare's works, Stephen Greenblatt draws on the phrase, 'the cunning of uncertainty',[34] used by historian of science Helga Nowotny to characterise such scientific fields as genetic engineering, big-data culturomics, economic modelling:

> it is a concept that perfectly characterises the fascination of Shakespeare and, specifically, the elusive and astonishing flexibility of the Shakespearean text. Each of his great plays is an adaptive, open system, complex, unfixed, and unpredictable. Shakespeare was the master of creative uncertainty and hence of ongoing, vital cultural mobility.[35]

Much the same applies to Keats. It is in this light, and with these terms in mind, that I wish to present Keats's *Lamia, Isabella, The Eve of St*

Agnes, And Other Poems (1820) as a 'multi-dimensional', unified work, At a more general level, I hope to show how, in a remarkable volume of poetry, the whole can exceed and enrich the constituent poems, revealing creative links between composition and publication, thus offering more general insight into the complex nature of creativity itself through the example of a poet consciously aware of his own 'self-canonisation', as one who claimed, 'that which is creative must create itself'.[36]

Melancholy: First Thoughts

I hope to show in Chapter 3 that there are various unifying stylistic and thematic elements which underly *1820*. In Chapters 4, 5 and 6, one overall theme in particular will be pursued. Analysis of the choice and ordering of poems, the collection can be read as mapping many paradoxical facets of the emotional ailment, melancholy. Deriving from its classical, Graeco-Roman roots, melancholy in the Renaissance was considered a serious and complex medical condition, inextricably connecting body and mind. It has not completely disappeared, since the clinical terrain of Renaissance melancholy has, in modern times, been transferred into psychology, incorporating mental conditions pathologised as anxiety, depression, mania, suicidal tendencies and a host of other serious disorders previously classified as facets of melancholy. In the eighteenth century it survived as a source for 'graveyard poetry' and Gothic novels, and for Romantics it became a fashionable poetic pose, which in Keats's time was rapidly palling in popular taste. All of these associations were known to Keats, and I hope to show in Chapter 6 that he drew upon each.

The existence of such a medically related preoccupation in *1820* is not surprising, since Keats was qualified as a surgeon-apothecary. Many scholars have shown how his training continued as a major influence on his poetry, providing references to specific medical states and remedies from the traditional and ever-expanding *materia medica* as a required course of study when Keats was a student.[37] He was also reading with great enthusiasm Burton's *Anatomy of Melancholy* during the period when he was putting together the collection, and this book was one of his favourites. It is recognised by Robert Gittings as a major influence on Keats's poetry in 1819.[38] The poems reveal a new set of interrelated meanings when seen as sequential reflections on different aspects of Renaissance and Romantic constructions of melancholy. It does not really matter to the argument whether Keats consciously planned this, since there is ample evidence that melancholy had long been at the forefront of his mind, both before and during the time when he came to plan the collection. From childhood, he also suffered from mood swings and bouts of melancholy himself.

Such a thematic approach to the 1820 volume seems also consistent with Keats's evolving, secular philosophy of the meaning of emotional suffering in a person's life, developed just at the time in April 1819 when he was writing some of the poems in the volume. He sees the journey of life as a 'vale of Soul-making' with the purpose of schooling the mind and intelligence into a soul as 'the seat of human Passions':

> Do you not see how necessary a World of Pains and troubles is to school an Intelligence and make it a soul? A Place where the heart must feel and suffer in a thousand ways? . . . This appears to me a faint sketch of a system of Salvation which does not affront our reason and humanity –.[39]

'Circumstances' of adversity and personal experiences are the key to an individuating process of 'Soul-making':

> I mean, I began by seeing how man was formed by circumstances – and what are circumstances? – but touchstones of his heart – ? And what are touchstones? – but proovings of his heart? – and what are proovings of his heart but fortifiers or alterers of his nature? And what is his altered nature but his soul? . . . And how is the heart to become this Medium but in a world of Circumstances? –

Keats is using 'proovings' in the contemporary medical sense (and still used thus in homeopathy), meaning 'testing, trialling' a drug to ascertain its effect on the mind or body.[40] It also bears a religious reference, to describe temptation as a formative test of faith, and part of Keats's aim is to construct a secular 'system of Salvation' as an alternative to the Christian 'vale of tears' (*valis lacrimarum, Psalm* 84 in some translations), excluding any presumption of original sin as the cause for human suffering. Keats's optimistic, humanistic view may have been forged in reaction against Wordsworth's bleaker allegory of growing away from the light: 'We Poets in our youth begin in gladness; | But thereof come in the end despondency and madness' ('Resolution and Independence', ll. 48–9). The word 'circumstances' in Keats's lexicon does not mean neutral, random occurrences in what he describes as 'the wide arable land of events', but a tangle of significant affective events, interspersing pleasure and pain, joy and melancholy, as he says in the same letter:

> This is the world – thus we cannot expect to give way many hours to pleasure – Circumstances are like Clouds continually gathering and bursting – While we are laughing the seed of some trouble is put into [the] wide arable land of events – while we are laughing it sprouts is [it] grows and suddenly bears a poison fruit which we must pluck – . . .[41]

This personal theory had roots in Keats's medical training. He is thinking and writing as a 'poet physician', though Brittany Pladek has advanced an important qualification, that he is also placing himself as 'patient as physician', generalising from his own personal experiences of emotional pain and suffering, viewed in the light of his medical training and his reading.[42] It is a subsidiary part of this book's design to suggest that the 1820 volume can be read as a poetic equivalent of the 'vale of Soul-making', where the poems themselves can be seen as 'circumstances' or 'proovings', stepping-stones through a vale of melancholy towards acceptance of its necessity in forming a unique soul, and in this case a unique volume.

Notes

1. Bate, *John Keats*, p. 650.
2. To Woodhouse, 27 October, 1818, *The Letters of John Keats 1814–1821* (hereafter *LJK*), 1, p. 387
3. Scott, 'Keats's American Ode', pp. 205–24.
4. Scott, 'Keats's American Ode', p. 206.
5. Blunden, *John Keats*, pp. 28–30.
6. Wasserman, *The Finer Tone: Keats' Major Poems* and Vendler, *The Odes of John Keats*.
7. Matthews, *Keats: The Critical Heritage*, pp. 123–32.
8. *Lamia, Isabella, The Eve of St Agnes 1820*. Facsimile.
9. Penguin Poetry First Editions, *Lamia, Isabella, The Eve of St Agnes and Other Poems*, with 'Note on the Text' by Michael Schmidt.
10. *Keats: Poems Published in 1820*, ed. M. Robertson.
11. Gittings, *John Keats: The Living Year*.
12. Stillinger, 'The Order of Poems in Keats's First Volume', pp. 1–13, 3.
13. Stillinger, *The Hoodwinking of Madeline*, p. 5.
14. Fraistat, *The Poem and the Book*, p. 98.
15. Fraistat, *The Poem and the Book*, p. 99.
16. Stillinger, 'Review', *Modern Philology*, 84 (May, 1987), pp. 436–7.
17. Fraistat (ed.), *Poems in Their Place: The Intertextuality and Order of Poetic Collections*, pp. 95–140.
18. Gamer, *Romanticism, Self-Canonization, and the Business of Poetry*, p. 2.
19. Greenblatt, *Renaissance Self-Fashioning: From More to Shakespeare*.
20. Gamer, *Romanticism, Self-Canonization, and the Business of Poetry*, p. 41.
21. To the George Keatses, 14–31 October, 1818, *LJK*, 1, p. 394.
22. This suggestion is offered by John Barnard in *John Keats: Selected Letters*, p. 246 fn.
23. Gamer, *Romanticism, Self-Canonization, and the Business of Poetry*, p. 33.
24. Tuve, *A Reading of George Herbert*, p. 152.
25. Gamer, *Self-Canonization, and the Business of Poetry*, ch. 4. See also Martz,

'George Herbert: The Unity of *The Temple*', which has in turn generated other studies along the same lines.

26. Fraistat, *Poems in their Place*, p. 1.
27. Earl Miner, 'Some Issues for the Study of Integrated Collections', in Fraistat, *Poems in their Place*, ch. 2.
28. *Milton's Sonnets*, ed. E. A. J. Honigmann, pp. 59–75.
29. Gill, *Wordsworth's Revisitings*, p. 14.
30. *The Complete Poems of D. H. Lawrence*, ed. Vivian de Sola Pinto and Warren Roberts, pp. 27–8.
31. *The Keats Circle* (hereafter *KC*), 2, p. 65.
32. Quoted from National Portrait Gallery archives, by Oliver Herford, 'Joseph Severn: On Likeness and Life-Writing', p. 320.
33. Harlan, 'Intellectual History and the Return of Literature', p. 598.
34. Nowotny, *The Cunning of Uncertainty*.
35. Greenblatt, 'King Lear, a difficult play, not helped by sloppy analysis'.
36. To James Hessey, 8 October, 1818, *LJK* 1, p. 374.
37. There are many studies of this subject, cited in Chapter 4.
38. Gittings, *John Keats: The Living Year*.
39. To George and Georgiana Keats, 21 April 1819, *LJK*, 2, p. 103.
40. For information about methods of distillation of medicines see Stuart Sperry, *Keats the Poet*.
41. *LJK*, 2, p. 79.
42. Pladek, *The Poetics of Palliation: Romantic Literary Therapy*, pp. 164–5.

*This is none of my doing — I w[as]
ill at the time.*

ADVERTISEMENT.

If any apology be thought necessary for the
appearance of the unfinished poem of HYPERION,
the publishers beg to state that they alone are
responsible, as it was printed at their particular
request, and contrary to the wish of the author.
The poem was intended to have been of equal
length with ENDYMION, but the reception given
to that work discouraged the author from proceeding. *This is a lie.*

Fleet-Street, June 26, 1820.

2.1 Keats's disclaimers scribbled on the 'Advertisement' in the presentation copy
to Burridge Davenport: Houghton Library at Harvard University, citation number
Keats *EC8.K2262.820l (G).

Chapter 2

Biography of a Book

In a meticulous study of the steps towards publication of Keats's first volume, *Poems 1817*, John Barnard analyses, in almost day by day detail, the progress towards publication of that earlier collection.[1] But very little comparable is offered by scholars on the 1820 volume, despite the fact that in terms of quality of poetry and as a monument in the history of the book, *1820* is undoubtedly more important than *Poems 1817* or *Endymion* (1818). Without claiming to be as thorough as Barnard, I summarise the main facts here.

It is possible to trace in general rather than specific details the writing and publication of Keats's collection which eventually appeared in 1820, its title page reading, 'LAMIA, ISABELLA, THE EVE OF ST AGNES, AND OTHER POEMS. | BY JOHN KEATS, AUTHOR OF ENDYMION | LONDON: PRINTED FOR TAYLOR AND HESSEY, 1820'.[2] Stung by the savage reviews and commercial failure of his previous efforts, *Poems* (1817) published on 10 March, 1817, and *Endymion: A Poetic Romance* published in early May, 1818, Keats was understandably disheartened when contemplating further publications. However, on 17 June 1819, he wrote to his sister Fanny,

> I was prepa[r]ing to enqu[i]re for a Situation with an Apothecary, put [*for* but] Mr Brown persuads [*sic*] me to try the press once more; so I will with all my industry and ability.[3]

By September 1819 he was, according to Woodhouse, writing to the publisher John Taylor, willing 'to publish the Eve of St Agnes & Lamia *immediately*: but Hessey told him it could not answer to do so now'.[4] At that stage he had decided against publishing 'Isabella' at all, thinking it 'mawkish', though Woodhouse disagreed. Already, Keats was quarrelling over some episodes in 'The Eve of St Agnes' with Woodhouse and, at second hand, Taylor, both of whom thought the explicit sexuality of Keats's revised version would deter women readers. This was an all-important consideration for the publishers, given their experience of how lucrative a middle-class female audience could be.[5] Perhaps over-reacting, Taylor wrote to Woodhouse:

> Had [Keats] known truly what the Society and what the Suffrages of Women are worth, he would never have thought of depriving himself of them. – So far as he is unconsciously silly in this Proceeding I am sorry for him, but for the rest I cannot but confess to you that it excites in me the Strongest Sentiment of Disapprobation.[6]

Perhaps he meant to write 'unconscionably' rather than 'unconsciously' but the strength of his feelings is clear enough. The publisher was also wary of provoking the kinds of critical attack made on the supposed prurience of *Endymion*. Taylor had his way and Keats retained the original version of 'The Eve', but the publisher's trials with the author were not over. Writing from Hampstead to Taylor, on 17 November, 1819, Keats wrote firmly, 'I have come to a determination not to publish any thing I have now ready written',[7] a corpus which by this time included all the poems which were to be included in *1820*. However, this did not mean an intention of abandoning his vocation as poet, since he goes on 'ambitiously' to plan out his career: 'but for all that to publish a Poem before long and that I hope to make a fine one'. Since he specifies 'a' single poem and claims, quoting from Milton's *Paradise Lost*, that 'the marvellous is the most enticing and the surest guarantee of harmonious numbers', it seems likely he had in mind returning to the *Hyperion* project, which he had first worked on from late 1818 to spring 1819 before abandoning this incomplete draft, taking it up again between July and September 1819 in a revision which he had again given up, at least temporarily. However, he is typically undecided about his plans ('I and myself cannot agree about this at all') and goes on to speak of writing 'Two or three' poems in which he wishes 'to diffuse the colouring of St Agnes eve throughout a Poem in which Character and Sentiment would be the figures to such drapery'. He hopes that writing such poems 'in the course of the next six years, would be a famous gradus ad Parnassum altissimum – ', adding, 'I mean they would nerve me up to the writing of a few fine Plays – my greatest ambition – when I do feel ambitious. I am sorry to say that is very seldom'.[8] He had already discussed with Taylor such a play, provisionally described as 'The Earl of Leicester's historry [sic]', based, like Shakespeare's history plays, on Holinshed's *Chronicles*. Some promising news arrived on 20 December that the play he had written jointly in a kind of Beaumont-and-Fletcher-like collaboration with Charles Brown, *Otho the Great*, was accepted by the Drury Lane theatre for production in the following spring, though this was never to eventuate.

Once again Taylor managed to talk Keats out of his reluctance to publish the volume of poems, or at least he may have overruled the poet and resolved to move ahead immediately, a courageous decision since they were still out of pocket over *Endymion*.[9] The definite decision to put together the 'Lamia' collection was made between the date of the letter to Taylor (17 November, 1819) and a relatively buoyant letter from John to his sister Fanny (written on 20 December, 1819). Keats reports the 'news but semigood' about *Otho* and declares 'My hopes of success in the literary world are now better than ever'. The crucial sentence from our point of view is this:

> I have been very busy since I saw you especially the last Week and shall be for some time, in preparing some Poems to come out in the S[p]ring and also in heightening the interest of our Tragedy [*Otho the Great*] . . .[10]

Ominously in the same letter to Fanny, whom he invariably protects by understating or concealing bad news, John also mentions having been 'unwell' and advised by his doctors to wear a new great coat and thick shoes, 'fearful le[s]t the weather should affect my throat which on exertion or cold continually threatens me . . .'. He promises to visit Fanny for Christmas but two days later says this is unlikely: 'I am sorry to say I have been and continue unwell'.[11] We can only wonder whether this dark medical subtext in a generally optimistic context may have created in Keats's mind a new urgency, inducing him to change his mind in deciding to collect 'some Poems to come out in the S[p]ring'. While continuing to remain optimistic about his health and to plan for the future, evidence from his medical training, the bitter experience of watching the decline and deaths of his mother and then his brother Tom (on 1 December, 1818), and his own anxiety in previously having to cut short his journeying with Brown in the north and Scotland because of a sore throat (August 1818), must all have planted seeds for doubt in his mind, especially with winter settling in. The fears deepened when, on 3 February 1819, he suffered a serious haemorrhage which was to keep him housebound for over a month and indirectly, after a series of 'nervous' letters to Fanny Brawne, led him to offer to break off their engagement.

Some progress in revising the poems seems to have been made during February, but on 8 March, 1820, Brown wrote with alarming news to Taylor: 'Poor Keats will be unable to prepare his Poe[e]ms for the Press for a long time. He was taken on Monday evening with violent palpitations at the heart, and has since remained too weak to get up'.[12] Two days later, however, Brown wrote again, more optimistically: 'After my dismal note I am glad to be able to give you good news. Keats is so well as to be out of danger', adding with barely credible hopefulness, that there is 'no organic defect whatever, – the disease is on his *mind*, and there I hope he will soon be cured'.[13] By 13 March Keats is back on the job preparing the volume, as Brown reports to Taylor:

> Keats has been slowly recovering; yesterday and to-day however he has been greatly altered for the better. He wishes his Poems to be published as soon as convenient to yourself, – the volume to commence with St Agnes Eve. He was occupied yesterday in revising Lamia. It is not his intention at present to have a Preface, – at least so we talked together to-day . . .'[14]

By 27 April, Taylor wrote to John Clare, whose first volume of poetry had been published by the same firm in January, 1820, that he has 'all Keats's MSS. in my hands now to make a Selection out of them for another volume'.[15] During this period, the collection may have been to the side of Keats's attention, judging from the distraught and emotionally volatile letters he was writing to Fanny Brawne. These make no mention of it, foregrounding instead the relationship now made so difficult by Keats's virtual quarantining from his love. He may not have been so closely engaged on the volume as if he were not ailing and distressed. Most of the publishers' revisions were marginal improvements,[16] but Laura E. Campbell has persuasively argued that in 'Ode to Psyche' their 'correction' of 'budded syrian' (which Keats wrote) to 'budded Tyrian' makes nonsense of the intended meaning by turning a flower into a dye.[17] Like most English poets, Keats did not get botanical details wrong.

From the first week of May, Charles Brown rented out the rooms in Wentworth Place, Hampstead, in order to take his annual summer journey to Scotland, and Keats had to move out, taking a room in 2 Wesleyan Place, Kentish Town. Without Brown as intermediary, Keats now had to negotiate directly with the publishers, Taylor and Hessey, and disputes ignited like grass fires between them. It is tantalisingly unclear who suggested what in regard to the contents and divisions in the 1820 volume, but there is evidence that there was a to-and-fro discussion going on. Jack Stillinger summarises:

> There are trial layouts of the title page pencilled near the front and again at the end of the W[1] book of transcripts: the one near the front has *Hyperion* as the second poem in the volume ("LAMIA | Hyperion, a Fragment, | ISABELLA | St. AGNES EVE, | and other poems"), and the one at the end, which may have been written earlier, omits *Hyperion* altogether ("Lamia; | Isabella; | The Eve of S[t] Agnes; | <with> | & Other poems | by | John Keats").[18]

Since the 'W[1] book of transcripts' refers to 'Transcripts in the smaller of two volumes of Woodhouse copies of poems at Harvard . . .' (Stillinger) it is possible that the notes may have been made by Woodhouse himself, who seems to have been the one most strongly in favour of including 'Hyperion'. In both 'layouts', 'Ode on Melancholy' could have been printed last in the volume. Even more intriguingly, Stillinger adds, 'Some pencil jottings on the verso of one of the leaves of the holograph fair copy of 'Lamia' suggest that the publishers at one time planned to issue each of the five sections of the volume as a separate pamphlet (see Lowell, II, p. 426, and Gittings, p. 401).'[19] These were to cost half-a-crown each. However, in the event the single, hard-bound volume was offered on sale at 7s.6d., 'cheap in my Opinion' wrote Taylor'.[20] In terms of the intended structure of *1820* the phrase 'each of the five sections of the volume' is tantalising, and they are specified as

1. Isabella
2. Lamia
3. St. Agnes
4. Poems. Miscellaneous
5. Hyperion. A fragment

Lowell concludes, 'the separate pamphlets were, it is evident, abandoned altogether, but one would like to know why they were ever contemplated'.[21] However, we might hypothesise that the publishers did not entirely 'abandon' the idea but gave themselves room for a possible future fall-back marketing strategy, by setting up each of the five sections with its own independent title page, making it easy by simply repaginating to re-issue them as pamphlets depending on sales. If so, Taylor and Hessey may have shrewdly anticipated today's 'print on demand' ploy of selling individual chapters of a book separately. It would also have left open a compromise solution to placate Keats, since if he had been able to complete a future *Hyperion* volume, the 'Fragment' could then simply be detached from copies of *1820*.

The weeks before publication were fraught ones for Keats. We find him 'tormented day and night' with love for Fanny Brawne, to whom he confides ominously that 'They talk of my going to Italy'.[22] He was still tidying up the proofs of his book, writing testily on 11(?) June to Taylor complaining about an apparently editorial change in 'St Agnes Eve': 'My meaning is quite destroyed in the alteration'.[23] Both his brother George and Haydon in the same week expressed concern at the news that John is 'very poorly'.[24] To Brown on about 21 June Keats says, 'My book (*Note) is coming out with very low hopes, though not spirits on my part. (*Note) Lamia, Isabella, The eve of Saint Agnes, and other poems.'[25] He is both laconic and frank in writing to his sister Fanny two days later:

I had intended to delay seeing you till a Book which I am now publishing was out, expecting that to be the end of this Week when I would have brought it to Walthamstow: on receiving your Letter of course I set myself to come to town, but was not able for just as I was setting out yesterday morning a slight spitting of blood came on which returned rather more copiously at night. I have slept well and they tell me there is nothing material to fear. I will send my Book soon with a Letter which I have had from George . . .[26]

The proofs of the poems themselves were finalised and presumably approved by Keats on about 11 June, but any satisfaction he may have felt must have quickly evaporated since on 22 June he haemorrhaged again. This induced him to move into Leigh Hunt's home, an arrangement which was to lead to domestic ructions and estrangement, fuelled by Keats's bouts of paranoia and panic, trapped as he felt in the enforced lack of privacy in the chaotic Hunt family environment. All in all, the whole period was marked by extreme distress and disruption for the poet. Nonetheless, on 26 June the volume was advertised and on Friday 30 June, 1820, Keats received forward copies of his book. It sold for seven shillings and sixpence. On the same day Hessey sent a copy to John Clare, so for want of more precise evidence that date can probably serve as a 'launch'[27] though Andrew Motion suggests 1 July.[28] On 1 July *The Literary Gazette* announced it was 'on the eve of publication', as noted by Reynolds who had evidently by then received his copy too: 'His Book looks like an angel & talks like one too'.[29] *Lamia, Isabella, The Eve of St Agnes, and Other Poems* was in print and in the public domain. The copy sent to Fanny Brawne (the headnote to Introduction), was rather coyly inscribed 'F. B. from J. K.', probably because Keats vowed not to publicise the relationship. It was, in Lowell's words, specially 'full bound in diamond-toothed calf, a habit of Keats's with very special copies of his various works'.[30] Taylor was extremely enthusiastic about the result: 'I am sure of this, that for Poetic Genius there is not his equal living, and I would compare him against anyone with either Milton or Shakespeare for Beauties'.[31] His partner Hessey was equally enthusiastic, writing to John Clare, 'For my own part I think no single volume of Poems ever gave me more real delight on the whole than I have received from this'.

However, Keats himself was not entirely pleased with the result, since some aspects of the publication did not meet his approval. He may have opened his first copy with mixed emotions of elation or apprehension, but in either case was met immediately with an 'Advertisement' written by the publishers explaining a difference of opinion between author and publishers:

Advertisement

If any apology be thought necessary for the appearance of the unfinished poem of HYPERION, the publishers beg to state that they alone are responsible, as it was printed at their particular request, and contrary to the wish of the author. The poem was intended to have been of equal length with ENDYMION, but the reception given to that work discouraged the author from proceeding.

Fleet Street, June 26 1820.

Woodhouse's initial draft of the Advertisement which he shared with Taylor said that the inclusion of 'the ensuing fragment' was 'not the wish of the author' but that the 'Publishers . . . prevailed upon him to allow of its form[ing] a part of this volume'.[32] It seems that they had not been able to 'prevail upon him' in reaching such an agreement, or at least not with equanimity. We do not need to speculate on Keats's reaction on opening the published work to see this, since we have clear evidence of what he felt. He was angry. The evidence lies in a presentation copy he sent to Burridge Davenport, a relatively wealthy merchant living 'at 2 Church Row in one of the two finest Georgian buildings in Hampstead',[33] an occasional dining partner whose wife had been especially solicitous of his brother Tom's health. Of Davenport, Keats had earlier written, 'We are to have a party this evening – the Davenports from Church row . . . they have paid me a good deal of attention – I like Davenport himself – ',[34] and later, 'Davenport from a sense of weakness thought it incumbent upon him to show off – and pursuant to that never ceased talking and boaring [boring? roaring?] all day, till I was completely fagged out – Brown grew melancholy . . .'.[35] In the copy of the book sent to Davenport, Keats crossed over all the Advertisement with double hatching and noted beside the reference to 'Hyperion. A Fragment', 'This is none of my doing – I w[as] ill at the time'. He bracketed the reference to *Endymion* and wrote against it, 'This is a lie'. The latter assertion is open to interpretation. What is the 'lie' in the publishers' statement? Was it 'The poem was intended to have been of equal length with ENDYMION', or 'but the reception given to that work discouraged the author from proceeding'? Is it the implication that the reception of *Endymion* had stopped Keats in his tracks while writing 'Hyperion', or the suggestion that he had not in fact been 'proceeding' with the latter? Both can be considered as at least seriously misleading if not outright 'lies', because Keats had been wrestling with a revised version in the three months before he decided to collect his poems for the 1820 volume. He seems to have discarded the earlier 'Hyperion' for stylistic reasons and because his approach to the myth had changed significantly in ways that created problems in providing a conclusion, neither of which had anything to do with the critical reception of *Endymion*. He had indeed 'proceeded' with the epic in all senses, and may still have intended to complete it, despite the hiatus caused by ill-health and the time spent putting together his 1820 collection. The second fragment was published long after his death as *The Fall of Hyperion. A Dream*. Amy Lowell who first published the denial wonders why it was on Davenport's copy only, and not on other presentation copies, such as Hazlitt's or Fanny Brawne's: 'For what reason Mr Davenport was singled out as the recipient of this unique confidence, we shall never know. Probably some conversation not recorded was the cause'.[36] This remains yet another mystery, but a couple of possible reasons suggest themselves. Other recipients may have already known of the circumstances and did not need reminding; or some copies may have been sent by the publishers from the author's list rather than the author himself. Besides, the 'Advertisement' is explicit enough not to require Keats's further disclaimer, which seems to have been written to Davenport on the spur of the moment and with impulsive anger. Of course, it is possible that Keats gradually calmed down, gratified at least to see his book in print.

One other possible reason for Keats's reluctance to include 'Hyperion' in the collection comes in a rather maddeningly gnomic and ambiguous comment by Reynolds writing to Milne long afterwards in 1848:

> I inclose you a letter of remonstrance, (which I found 28 years old! amongst the originals of Keats's Letters) against the printing the marvellous fragment of Hyperion with a work of Leigh Hunt. I longed to get him free from being a Political adherent to a good, though then dangerous Side for a young Poet.[37]

It is not clear whose is the 'remonstrance', whether on the side of Reynolds or Keats, but Reynolds seems to be saying he was trying to persuade Keats 'against the printing of the marvellous fragment of Hyperion with a work of Leigh Hunt', suggesting that he was trying to prise Keats away from the influence of Hunt and the older poet's political association. If the letter was '28 years old!' in 1848 then it would have been written in 1820, but by then Keats had weaned himself off Hunt's poetic influence (though he continued to be personally indebted to him, even as a guest in Hunt's house) and the 'danger' may have abated, so much had Keats's own style matured into independence. Even allowing for Reynolds' increasingly intense dislike for Hunt,[38] he was probably right that the perception of closeness between Hunt and Keats by hostile reviewers would have been triggered, as it had been on publication of *Poems 1817* and *Endymion*. Further puzzles are whether Reynolds is referring to the first or second 'fragment of Hyperion', both of which were in existence, and also what the projected 'work of Leigh Hunt' was. Too many mysteries enshroud Reynolds' tantalising comment to build any argument upon, and unfortunately the letter he refers to is not in existence, or at least not published. Stillinger adds one more detail to the jigsaw: 'J. H. Reynolds's "remonstrance" against 'printing ... Hyperion with a work of Leigh Hunt' is corroborated by the fact that Hunt possessed Keats's holograph'.[39] This apparently explains why Woodhouse's transcript was used as copy for the published text, which in turn adds evidence that the decision was entirely that of the publishers, and that Hunt could not be persuaded to part with Keats's holograph. It may not be entirely fanciful to hypothesise that Hunt, with typical generosity, may have been trying to help mediate a *contretemps* between Keats and the publishers by making the compromise suggestion of a separate, jointly-authored volume. He may have judged that Keats was not necessarily averse to publishing the fragment, but just not in the 1820 volume, and if Hunt was the one who made the offer, he might have been trying to get around this problem.

However we may interpret the 'lie', the phrase 'This is none of my doing' is unambiguously forthright and accords with the wording of the 'Advertisement' itself – 'contrary to the wishes of the author'. It is also consistent with Woodhouse's draft formulation ('not the wish of the author'). In other words, whether or not Keats was finally persuaded, however reluctantly, to approve the inclusion of the 'Hyperion' fragment in the collection, yet he clearly remained neither happy nor reconciled, at least in private. His clear preference was to end the volume with 'Ode on Melancholy', and this is the assumption I will be building upon, in terms of the plan behind his choice of poems and their ordering, and in asserting the integrity and unity of the whole. In my earlier book, *John Keats: A Literary Life*, I briefly sketched a hypothesis of the fraught psychological and emotional situation faced by Keats himself and his publishers from their different perspectives, and I see no reason to withdraw from it:

> Equally objectionable must have been the choice of the earlier and discarded *Hyperion. A Fragment* despite the existence of the later, more mature *The Fall of Hyperion. A Dream.* Even the latter was clearly not the end of Keats's aspiration since during 1820 he several times repeated his plan to continue and complete the poem about Hyperion. Epic was always his litmus test for greatness in non-dramatic poetry, and the form he aspired to. One can see his point. The publishers' decision, however well-meaning, looks like an anticipation that the poet would not live to publish a long poem in a single volume like *Endymion*, and however realistic this may have been, it can be seen as singularly insensitive, almost a prediction of his inevitable death.[40]

Meiko O'Halloran attributes Keats's determination to turn away from the mode of pastoral in *Endymion* and towards an epic comparable to Milton's *Paradise Lost*, to his visit to Staffa and Fingal's Cave on his northern walking tour in July 1818. Here, by internalising the emotional suffering in Milton's elegy *Lycidas*, he found his own motivation for a transition into the realm of the epic.[41] It was to become more rather than less important to him as time went on. The publishers' decision to publish prematurely, and present a discarded or superseded draft, may have contributed to his 'habitual feeling' expressed in November 1820, that he was already 'leading a posthumous existence'.[42] His declaration to Reynolds that he was abandoning the project on 21 September, 1819, seems only to refer to what he has already written, especially since the reason he gives refers to a specific stylistic point that it is too 'Miltonic'. Jeffrey Cox notes that there is some evidence that 'he may have made some revisions in November–December 1819',[43] suggesting he had taken it up again. Everybody was worried about Keats's ill-health, even the poet himself, but the signs are that he was not yet ready to 'put his affairs in order' and was still focused on future plans. These included even giving up writing poetry altogether, in favour of paid journal essays and theatre reviews, or alternatively, in his words in the very month he was proofreading *1820*, 'I shall try what I can do in the Apothecary line',[44] or becoming a ship's doctor on an Indiaman vessel. However, the thought of returning to medicine seems to have been a desperate measure and elsewhere he discards the idea.

He still had much to live for. His doctors, perhaps more in protective hope than conviction, were encouraging of a recovery, he had the prospect of seeing *Otho the Great* performed at Drury Lane or Covent Garden with, he still hoped, Edmund Kean starring. He seems to have had a fairly clear authorial 'career path' in mind, of alternating collections of short poems (*1817* and *1820*) with volumes containing a single long poem, an epic (*Endymion* and later *Hyperion*). To draw a comparison, it is quite common for writers of prose fiction to alternate collections of short stories and full-length novels, for a variety of reasons from the commercial to the artistic.[45] 'Hyperion' was clearly intended to be next off the blocks after his 1820 collection depending on its reception, and he had already an advanced second draft to work with. He had forecast this intention in his preface to *Endymion*: 'I hope I have not in too late a day touched the beautiful mythology of Greece, and dulled its brightness; for I wish to try once more, before I bid it farewel.' Why would he wish to spike or distort the chances of the ambitious, future epic by publishing an early, fragmentary, and already discarded 'false start', particularly since his use of the myth had changed radically even between the two versions, as his vision had matured so rapidly? It seems to make both intuitive and biographical sense that, until he felt he had completed to his own satisfaction a long poem based on the Hyperion myth, he would not wish any version to be placed before the public. In terms of his 'career path' he had already proved he could write a play, which he saw as his destined 'gradus ad Parnassum altissimum', and he had begun in August 1819 writing another, a tragedy of *King Stephen*. Since he already had a lot on his plate, it may not be quite so accurate to say, as Stillinger does, that he 'abandoned' the whole 'Hyperion' project: Barnard's more cautious 'put it aside' seems to ring more true. There is evidence within the incomplete draft that he had some problems to solve about the ordering of the narrative in its second half of a projected four parts. He had yet other plans, having also begun and part-published a poem completely unlike his other published works, the satirical *The Cap and Bells; or, The Jealousies. A Faery Tale*, using a female *nom de plume*, Lucy Vaughan Lloyd. A rather puzzling work in Keats's canon as a kind of *jeu d'esprit*, it may have been an attempt to capture and exploit a market for rakish Regency smartness, and signals a new, original direction in his writing. In short, Keats had a lot to look forward to in his chosen profession as poet, and no reason to authorise publication of an unfinished, discarded version of his next projected poem of epic proportions, 'Hyperion'. He was certainly not ready to die, and in his mind his journey through the 'vale of Soul-making' was not done.

If part of the thinking of Woodhouse, Taylor and Hessey was that Keats would not live to see his future publishing plans fulfilled, they turned out to be tragically correct. Admittedly also, virtually all reviewers and poets at the time, whether grudgingly or enthusiastically, singled out the fragment as qualitatively different and of a higher order than the other poems, so if it had not been published in *1820* contemporaries would have missed its grandeur and sublimity altogether. In this sense, the publishers deserve gratitude, since a version of *The Fall of Hyperion. A Dream* was not published until long after his death. Whether their collective judgment was also right in thinking 'Hyperion. A Fragment' belongs in this particular collection on thematic and aesthetic grounds, is a different and open question to which we shall return in the last chapter. For the time being, I proceed on the working hypothesis that the book Keats himself envisaged would have ended with 'Ode on Melancholy', and that its unity can be analysed on this basis.

If Keats had chosen, like Lawrence, to present the poems in chronological order of composition, it would have looked something like this (with some uncertainty about the exact date of 'Psyche'), the order in which most modern editions present the poems, interspersed with others:

Robin Hood
Lines on the Mermaid Tavern

Isabella; or, The Pot of Basil
Fancy
Bards of Passion and of Mirth
The Eve of St Agnes
Hyperion. A Fragment
Ode to Psyche
Ode to a Nightingale
Ode on a Grecian Urn
Ode on Indolence
Lamia
To Autumn

If nothing else, this order would have highlighted the rapid and dramatic development of the poet's craft. This seems to have been at least one consideration which Keats wanted to signal in his first collection, *Poems* (1817), where he wrote in a preliminary note, 'THE short Pieces in the middle of the Book, as well as some of the Sonnets, were written at an earlier period than the rest of the Poems'. The order in that volume had not been systematically chronological, but by mentioning that some were 'written at an earlier period' he perhaps hoped that the volume's quality would be judged on the poems written later, and with an eye to future improvement. This seems not an issue in compiling *1820*.

As published, the poems in *1820* are presented in the following order, with gaps indicating each section which has its individual title page (signalled in the list below in italics). The arrangement first suggests a formal grouping into different genres:

Lamia
Isabella
The Eve of St Agnes
POEMS
Ode to a Nightingale
Ode on a Grecian Urn
Ode to Psyche
Fancy
Ode ['Bards of passion and of mirth']
Lines on the Mermaid Tavern
Robin Hood
To Autumn
Ode on Melancholy
Hyperion. A Fragment

These are certainly not in chronological order of composition. The three romances may have been adjudged the volume's main commercial attraction, given the contemporary fashion for their genre, especially among the women readers Taylor and Woodhouse were keen not to offend. These are followed by 'Poems', which include a group of brief, more comic lyrics, in turn framed by odes. In other words, genre itself is not the only principle of ordering. Odes are not grouped as a generic block, since 'Nightingale', 'Grecian Urn' and 'Psyche' are separated from 'Autumn' and 'Melancholy', while 'Ode' ('Bards of Passion and of Mirth') is placed with the *'rondeaux'*. This further suggests a deliberate but different, sequential arrangement of the material, such as thematic development of thought or internal cohesion. The odes are self-reflective and intellectually playful discussions of art, music, and poetry, all linked by the capacity of the imagination to deceive and, like love, create illusions which subvert rational thought. Musical art itself is likened to a form of madness that brings the persona in 'Ode to a Nightingale' close to ecstatic suicide, and the 'plaintive' and 'forlorn' mood caused by its cessation is a form of melancholy picked up in other poems. These themes had surfaced in the longer, opening poems, and the shorter poems comment on them in an implicitly interrogative mood, as though the odes are self-consciously analysing the kind of art that the previous, longer poems represent.

Another possible choice for the adopted ordering is based on a historical timeline for their respective settings, sources, and authorial stance. 'Lamia' recounts a story from classical mythology; 'Isabella' is a Medieval story from Boccaccio; and 'The Eve of St Agnes' draws on Renaissance sources, Shakespeare's *Romeo and Juliet* and Burton's *The Anatomy of Melancholy*. It is also the kind of neo-Gothic tale popular in Romantic-age novels such as Ann Radcliffe's. The group which follows, having their own internal 'title page' as 'Poems', are essentially lyrics spoken in the present tense. After reflecting on the past in 'Ode on a Grecian Urn' and 'Ode to Psyche', lamenting the loss of Elizabethan poets and Robin Hood, they bring the collection up to the poet's simultaneous temporal present with 'To Autumn', which itself is lined with an elegiac tone conceding the passing of time. 'Ode on Melancholy' is pitched as a generalising, mythic present, comparable to the effect of the final two sonnets in Shakespeare's sequence (153 and 154). I would be fascinated to know if Keats hesitated over whether to place 'Ode to a Nightingale' before 'To Autumn' as the only other lyric poem located in the simultaneous present, but as I shall argue in Chapter 6, its affinities in sources, imagery, and ambivalent closure lie more with 'The Eve of St. Agnes'.

As in other ways, 'Hyperion. A Fragment' would break such a sequence by returning to classical mythology, making it appear even more like an 'Appendix' to the collection. It finishes without any pretence of closure, mid-line and in the middle of a sentence, in a way which implies (probably truthfully) that the poet did not quite know where it was headed:

> Apollo shriek'd; – and lo! from all his limbs
> Celestial * * * * * *
> * * * * * * * *

THE END.

Nothing could be further removed from the effect which would be achieved of elegant closure in the last lines of 'Ode on Melancholy', which does provide a unity and thematic completion to a studied sequence of thought, while also inviting retrospective reflection, synthesis, and reinterpretation of the earlier poems. It is also the only poem in the collection to gesture in its final, beautiful lines towards a posthumous future for both the poet and his volume: 'His soul *shall taste* the sadness of her might, |And *be among* her trophies *hung*' (my italics).

Reception of the volume was more positive than that for his two earlier books. Several reviews appeared during July, August and September, and as was customary in the politically internecine world of journals at the time, they divided along partisan lines, with Keats's friends, Lamb, Hunt and Barry Cornwall leading the cheer squad. Former critics were more qualified or silent this time around. The blazoning in *1820* of *Endymion* on the title page and in the 'Advertisement' was risky and audacious to the point of provocation, given the storm of notoriety around that poem generated by the negative and offensively personal attacks, on the 'Cockney School of Poetry' by John Gibson Lockhart, signing himself 'Z', in *Blackwood's Magazine* (August 1818), and by John Wilson Croker (though reputedly written by the editor, William Gifford), in *Quarterly Review* (September 1818). These were malicious and hurtful pieces, though their real target was not Keats himself but Leigh Hunt. What had made these earlier Tory attacks especially effective was that they went unanswered in the Whig press, represented by the *Edinburgh Review*. Its editor, Francis Jeffrey, 'the most influential and respected critic of the day', seemed to have this on his conscience, since on the appearance of *1820* he published a lengthy and appreciative review of *Endymion* which he may have penned in 1818, adding at the end a very brief but positive notice of the later volume, claiming to have 'left ourselves room to say but little of the second volume'.[46] Much later on 15 August 1818, he wrote to R. Monckton Milnes, 'I never regretted anything more than to have been *too late* with my testimony to [Keats's] merits'.[47] Meanwhile, there were enough positive reviews of the 1820 volume to forestall criticism, by anonymous writers in the *Monthly Review*, *Guardian*, *London Magazine and Monthly Critical and Dramatic Review*, *New Monthly Magazine* and *Monthly Magazine*. Carping criticism, damning with faint praise, came from *Eclectic Review* and three others. But on the whole the reception of this volume was more positive than that of the previous two, enough to please the publishers and author, if he had not by that time been too ill to appreciate it.

Not that the favourable notices did much to help sales, so entrenched had become the earlier deprecations in the reading public's estimation. At first, things seemed to be going well and he wrote to Charles Brown on 14 August, 'My book has had good success among literary people, and, I believe, has a moderate sale'.[48] However, on the very same day Taylor wrote to John Clare, 'We have some Trouble to get through 500 Copies of [Keats's] Work, though it is highly spoken of in the periodical Works'.[49] Just a few days later Keats himself was to report to Brown,

> The sale of my book is very slow, though it has been very highly rated. One of the causes, I understand from different quarters, of the unpopularity of this new book, and the others also, is the offence the ladies take at me.[50]

The last phrase may be more sarcastic than sincere, recalling his quarrels with the publishers over 'St. Agnes Eve'. Taylor may not have resiled from his belief in the high quality of the book, but he had grown somewhat pessimistic about the commercial realities, especially since 'the house had been sailing dangerously close to insolvency'.[51] His pessimism was based not only on lagging sales but also on a recognition that any potential interest in a new book of poetry was immediately swallowed by the distraction of a more sensational headline news of a royal scandal. (Nothing changes in the British popular press.) Even ten years later in 1830 the stock was not sold out, though at least expenses had been covered. On 11 September, 1820, Taylor wrote a legalistic and businesslike 'explicit Statement' to Keats, spelling out the terms under which he and Hessey had published the volume. He pointedly reminds the poet that they had not yet made a profit on *Endymion*, and reports that 'Lamia has not yet repaid the Expenses'.[52] However, Taylor touchingly stresses that they genuinely have the poet's welfare at heart and will continue to publish his poems: 'I hope yet to see you as rich and as renowned as you deserve to be'. Despite his stern tone, the financial arrangement Taylor proposed to Keats was magnanimous, and took into account the decision that the poet was so ill that he would have to go to the warmer climate of Italy. However, as late as 9 January 1835, Taylor was to write with sad resignation, 'I should like to print a complete

Edition of Keats's Poems, but the world cares nothing for him – I fear that even 250 copies would not sell'.[53] On 17–18 September 1820, both Taylor and Woodhouse sailed with Keats, Severn and Haslam on the *Maria Crowther* as far as Gravesend (tragic symbolism in the name). This was the last time they were to see the poet in whom they had invested such generous financial support and unflagging hope.

*

As a brief, more positive postscript, we might note that Keats's wish to 'be among the English Poets after my death' came, at least in a manner of speaking, more rapidly and unexpectedly than anybody could have expected. The ever-loyal Leigh Hunt in 1821 provided his sister-in-law, Elizabeth Kent, with information[54] towards a book she was compiling, entitled *Flora Domestica, or The Portable Flower-Garden*, to be published by Taylor and Hessey in 1823. Despite the publishers' misgivings, it seems to have been successful enough to warrant a second edition just two years later.[55] Kent presents her work as a catalogue of plants in alphabetical order, from Adonis and African Lily through to Winter Cherry and Zinnia. True to her subtitle *Illustrations from the Works of the Poets*, Kent provides quotations from a wide variety of poets both ancient and modern, to 'illustrate' the appearance, properties and symbolism of the plants. In this veritable anthology of the poetry of florilegia, she includes many sections from Keats's poetry, so that he appears alongside the likes of writers such as Ovid, Virgil, Petrarch, Ariosto, Boccaccio, Chaucer, Spenser, Sidney, Shakespeare, Milton, Davenant, Cowper, Campbell, Wordsworth, Shelley, Clare and a host of others: if not all 'English Poets' certainly illustrious ones. A generous number of Keats quotations adorn the items on Basil (of course), Clematis, Convolvulus, Laburnum, Fox-Glove, Hawthorn, Hyacinth, Marigold, Narcissus, Primrose, Rose, Sweet-Pea, Violet, and Water-lily. The aptly named Daisy Hay has argued plausibly that Leigh Hunt in his collaboration had an ulterior motive behind the selection, not only rehabilitating Keats against the attacks, but also promoting his 'Cockney School' poets and generally inserting politically charged statements into Kent's prose.[56] Inclusion of a generous selection of Keats's quotations may be a product of subtle special pleading 'in the family', but nonetheless represents a modest, swift and auspicious enlistment of Keats into the ranks of the poetic immortals.

Notes

1. Barnard, 'First Fruits or "First Blights', pp. 71–93.
2. This reproduces the punctuation used by Keats on his title page, and I reproduce quotations from this volume.
3. To Fanny Keats, 17 June 1819, *LJK*, 2, p. 121.
4. Woodhouse to Taylor, 19, 20 September 1819, *KC*, 1, pp. 90–1.
5. Chilcott, A *Publisher and his Circle*, p. 41.
6. Taylor to Woodhouse, 25 September 1819, *LJK*, 2, p. 183.
7. To John Taylor, 17 November 1819, *LJK*, 2, p. 234.
8. To Taylor, 17 November 1819, *LJK*, 2, p. 234.
9. Chilcott, p. 45.
10. To Fanny Keats, 20 December 1820, *LJK*, 2, pp. 236–8.
11. Ibid. p. 238.
12. Brown to Taylor 10 March 1820, *LJK*, 2, p. 274; *KC*, 1, p. 104.
13. Ibid. *LJK*, 2, pp. 274–5.
14. Brown to Taylor, 13 March 1820, *LJK*, 2, p. 276; *KC*, 1, p. 105.
15. Quoted Blunden, *London Mercury*, p. 141; attribution by Stillinger, *The Texts of Keats's Poems*, p. 67.
16. Gittings, *The Odes of Keats and their Earliest Known Manuscripts*, p. 71.
17. Laura E. Campbell, pp. 53–8.
18. Stillinger (ed.), *The Poems of John Keats*.
19. Ibid. p. 737.
20. Gittings, *John Keats*, p. 401.
21. Lowell, 2, p. 426.
22. To Fanny Brawne, *LJK* 2, p. 303. Rollins dates this 5 July 1820, but Gittings proposes May, and Barnard more recently, 'May/early June 1820'.
23. To Taylor, 11 June 1820, *LJK*, 2, p. 294.
24. From George Keats, 18 June 1820, *LJK*, 2, p. 296.
25. To Brown, about 21 June 1820, *LJK*, 2, p. 298.
26. To Fanny Keats, 23 June 1820, *LJK*, 2, p. 300.
27. See *LJK*, 2, p. 300, footnote 2.
28. Motion, *Keats*, p. 521.
29. Reynolds to Taylor, 3 July 1820, *KC*, 1, p. 120.
30. Lowell, 2, p. 426.
31. The letter, apparently lost, quoted by Lowell 'from Sir Sidney Colvin's *Life of Keats*, from information supplied by a great-niece of Taylor's'; Lowell, 2, p. 427.
32. Woodhouse, June, 1820, *KC*, 1, pp. 115–16.
33. To Mrs Burridge Davenport, November 1820, *LJK*, 1, p. 408 fn 1.
34. To George Keatses, 13 March 1819, *LJK* 2, pp. 76–7.
35. To George Keatses, 15 April 1819, *LJK*, 2, p. 83.
36. Lowell, 2, p. 425.
37. Taylor to Woodhouse, March, 1821, *KC*, 2, p. 234, fn 2.
38. Reynolds, *The Letters of John Hamilton Reynolds*, pp. xxviii–xxix.
39. Stillinger, *The Texts of Keats's Poems*, p. 230. See also Barnard, 'Manuscripts and Publishing History', p. 75 and note 1.
40. R. S. White, *John Keats: A Literary Life*, rev. edn, p. 217.

41. O'Halloran, May 2019 eprint.
42. To Brown, 30 November, 1820, *LJK*, 2, p. 359.
43. Jeffrey Cox, *Keats's Poetry and Prose*, p. 497.
44. To Taylor, 11 June, 1820, *LJK*, 2, p. 294.
45. A relevant example might be the output of the great Irish fiction writer, John McGahern.
46. Matthews, pp. 202–9.
47. Matthews, p. 209.
48. To Brown, 14 August 1820, *LJK*, 2, p. 321.
49. Quoted Edmund Blunden, *Keats's Publisher*, pp. 111–12.
50. To Brown, August(?), 1820, *LJK*, 2, p. 327.
51. Chilcott, p. 52.
52. Taylor to Keats, 11 September 1820, *KC,* 1, p. 138.
53. Blunden, *Keats's Publisher*, p. 190.
54. Letter from Hunt to Kent from Genoa dated 15 June 1822, <http://digital.lib.uiowa.edu/cdm/compoundobject/collection/leighhunt/id/944/rec/11> (last accessed 23 March 2020)
55. Kent, *Flora Domestica*
56. Hay, pp. 272–80.

Chapter 3

Multidimensional Unity: 'A Dozen Features of Propriety'

On 10–11 May 1817, Keats wrote to Benjamin Haydon:

> I remember your saying that you had notions of a good Genius presiding over you – I have of late had the same thought for things which [I] do half at Random are afterwards confirmed by my judgment in a dozen features of Propriety – Is it too daring to Fancy Shakspeare this presider?[1]

The phrase, 'things which [I] do half at Random are afterwards confirmed by my judgment in a dozen features of Propriety', brilliantly encapsulates a recognition that surely can be affirmed by any serious and original artist. The process of composition can appear semi-automatic, 'half at Random'; an act of writing which is delivered in the full engagement of the imagination when the writer is 'in the zone', to use a common modern phrase. Yet *ex post facto* critical rereadings may reveal patterns and 'features of Propriety' which were not consciously recognised or planned at the time of writing. Keats himself gives a complementary clue about his habits of composition in saying elsewhere of 'Ode to Psyche', 'I have for the most part dash'd of[f] my lines in a hurry – This I have done leisurely – I think it reads the more richly for it . . .'.[2] 'Dash'd of[f] my lines in a hurry' accords with 'half at Random', while in 'Psyche' he seems to have exercised the reflective rereading as he went along. Generally speaking, Keats composed with facility and spontaneity when the poem was ready to come 'as naturally as the Leaves to a tree',[3] even when he was laboring mightily, as in the task of writing *Endymion*. Unlike some of his contemporaries, when Keats made changes they were tinkerings, excisions and verbal embroidering, rather than full scale revisions (with the exception of the 'Hyperion' fragments). As Stillinger notes, 'Manuscript after manuscript shows him getting *most* of the words right the first time. And for all the textual and biographical materials at our disposal, we really don't have the faintest idea how he managed to do this'.[4] The distinction Keats himself draws is one between different functions, the first practised by the writer *as writer* while composing, and the second by the writer *as reader*, standing back from the work and analysing it in a more distanced, critical light. The writer is the first discriminating reader of his own work. In this chapter I look at how this might be exemplified in *1820*, both in individual poems and the whole volume, providing overlapping and reinforcing interconnected layers to the collection as a whole. 'A dozen features of Propriety' emerges as a multidimensional understanding of unity that allows the whole to transcend the parts in a collection which has its own internal integrity.

1. Enchantment and Disenchantment

Let us take Fraistat's main thematic concentration as the first of our 'dozen features' recurring in the volume. As his account develops, the recurrent and dominant pattern he finds is primarily thematic, a concentration on enchantment followed by disenchantment. This operates in at least some of the poems if not equally in all. In the romances pairs of lovers are 'undone' by love, and enchantment gives way to disillusionment (which Fraistat links with Shakespeare's *Troilus and Cressida* which Keats was reading at the time). The argument applies in obvious ways to 'Lamia' and 'Isabella' but is perhaps less convincing for 'The Eve of St Agnes', if we read that poem as one of liberation from family constrictions, surpassing Madeline's initial awakening from dream to reality. The conclusion could be seen as ending on disenchantment with the deaths of Angela and the Beadsman, but also as the start of a new life for the lovers. Next, the famous odes can be seen to be built upon the capacity of the imagination to enchant, presented as at war with the insufficiency of the imaginative fictions to overcome suffering and being forced, in Fraistat's words, to 'face the consequences of disenchantment'.[5] Again, however, while applying clearly to 'Nightingale' it is arguably less helpful in interpreting any of the other odes. The short poem 'Fancy', which Fraistat locates 'at the exact center' of the volume (since he sees the inclusion of 'Hyperion' as finally approved by Keats), provides a transition from enchantment as a falsifying quality, to one which has its own autonomous logic. In Fraistat's reading the apparently lightweight mid-poems crucially move from fancy to imagination, turning to the celebration of 'the imagination's power to study the human heart and mind' in the hands of the old poets in 'the larger, more heroic vision of the past' (p. 131). The poems that follow, Fraistat argues, form an antithesis to the earlier ones: 'Thus, unlike "The Eve of

St Agnes", "To Autumn" is a poem that confronts, rather than retreats from, a world of process and loss' (p. 130), resisting enchantment, while 'Ode on Melancholy' also asks the 'compelling question' whether the mind can 'sustain the burdens of disenchantment and loss?' which is seen as then being taken up in 'Hyperion'. With some qualifications, then, let us accept enchantment and disenchantment' as one of our 'features of Propriety' working to link the poems.

2. Dreams and Visions

Running alongside enchantment and disenchantment, references to dreams and visions recur, at least in the first half of the volume. In 'Lamia' they are especially prominent and ambiguous, as though acting as a vehicle 'To unperplex bliss from its neighbour pain'. 'Dream' occurs eleven times in this poem, and although the word 'vision' is not used, yet the transformed lamia is by definition a 'vision' rather than a woman. Hermes appears to Lamia in a 'splendid dream': 'I dreamt I saw thee, robed in purple flakes . . .', and offers Hermes a glimpse of the 'wood-nymph' he desires:

It was no dream; or say a dream it was,
Real are the dreams of Gods, and smoothly pass
Their pleasures in a long eternal dream.

A kind of paradoxical relativity is invoked in the dreamtime existence of immortals, since everything that happens in their realm is at once both dream and not-dream, since 'Real are the dreams of Gods'. Lamia herself 'dreams when in the serpent prison-house, | Of all she lists, strange and magnificent', and while 'dreaming thus' she sees the young Corinthian Lycius for the first time. The fatal ambiguity of the mutually sustained dream of love is intuited by Lycius on seeing his 'trusty guide' the sage Apollonius: 'but to-night he seems | The ghost of folly haunting my sweet dreams'. It is to be this figure who does indeed shatter his dream by penetrating the lamia's assumed appearance as a woman, revealing this to be a different kind of deceptive dream.

Just as fatefully, in the next poem Isabella sees her murdered lover in a kind of dream: 'His image in the dusk she seem'd to see' (stanza XXX) and later in a ghostly visitation: 'It was a vision. – In the drowsy gloom, | The dull of midnight, at her couch's foot | Lorenzo stood, and wept' (stanza XXXV). The 'pale shadow' tells her where the slain body is to be found. Next, in 'The Eve of St Agnes' the premonitory dream is central to the myth of St Agnes' night, though in the poem we are not told of its content: 'Shaded was her dream | By the dusk curtains: – 'twas a midnight charm | Impossible to melt as iced stream' (stanza XXXII), followed by the repetition of 'melt', this time made 'possible': 'Into her dream he melted, as the rose | Blendeth its odour with the violet, – | Solution sweet' (stanza XXXVI). Madeline is awakened in a fashion that has aroused differing interpretations as to whether the dream is a harbinger of joy or an ominous violation of innocence, an ambiguity which is embedded in a sequence of contrasting imagery. In these three poems, then, dreams are centrally functional to the narrative and also deeply ambivalent in meaning. Their uncertain doubleness resurfaces in the dazed state which concludes 'Ode to a Nightingale': 'Was it a vision, or a waking dream? Fled is that music: – Do I wake or sleep?', and again in 'Ode to Psyche': 'Surely I dreamt to-day, or did I see | The winged Psyche with awaken'd eyes?'. True or false, real or unreal, benign or menacing, it seems that in the 1820 volume dreams are at least problematical in terms of their truth-telling value.

3. Loss

Loss, traditionally considered a major trigger for melancholy, is also a central preoccupation running through Keats's poems in *1820*, occurring to a greater or lesser extent and in different contexts in all the poems. So insistent is the motif that, in each case, the poem's existence itself is offered as part compensation for the loss enacted in it. In 'Lamia', Lycius loses his love and finally his life, when his perception of the serpent change-ling's beauty is punctured by the clear-sighted philosopher, Apollonius, revealing the deception. At the same time, Lamia, whose love for Lycius is indeed sincere, also loses her love, as well as her temporary life as a woman. 'Isabella; or, The Pot of Basil' is a tale of unrelenting tragic loss, as Lorenzo is murdered and the chain of events lead to Isabella pining and eventually dying in grief. In 'The Eve of St Agnes' the central event is the loss of Madeline's virginity, which may be a 'fortunate fall' since it leads her away from her repressive family and allows her to escape 'into the storm' of independence with her lover: 'and they are gone – ay, ages long ago | These lovers fled away into the storm'. The final victims of the transition are the two aged figures who have been like benign guardians to her, Angela and the Beadsman, the first of whom dies 'palsy-twitched' while the latter ambiguously 'unsought for slept among his ashes cold'. Meanwhile, each of the shorter 'Poems' which follow contemplates dif-ferent kinds and degrees of loss, eliciting different poetic responses. The odes chart aspects of loss, such as the fading of music in 'Nightingale', inability to retrieve fully the past in 'Grecian Urn', and in 'Autumn' the gradual loss of summer days of warm fruition and autumnal routines. Meanwhile, 'Psyche' optimistically seeks to reverse the loss of pre-Olympian mythology by establishing a place for her in the classical canon. In 'Lines on the Mermaid Tavern' we have the refrain 'Poets dead and gone'; in 'Bards of Passion and of Mirth' (named simply 'Ode'), 'the souls ye left behind you | Wisdom, though fled far away'. Cultural loss is charted in 'Robin Hood', again emphasised in its refrain, 'No! those days are gone away, | Gone . . .'; and in 'Fancy', 'beauties that the earth hath lost | At a touch sweet Pleasure melteth | Pleasure never is at home'. 'Ode on Melancholy' offers another evaluation of loss, as its fleeting, intense evanescence is hailed as *carpe diem* (Horace, Book 1, Song 11). 'Hyperion: A Fragment' also dwells on loss as the irrevocable emotional state of the defeated Titans, though coming after 'Autumn' and 'Melancholy', this seems out of place in the volume as a backward step.

While some of these examples suggest something may be gained while something is lost, yet the reasoning turns on loss itself as the leading emotional event in each poem. Writers on melancholy, from the Renaissance Robert Burton through to the father of modern psychiatry Sigmund Freud, emphasised loss as a primary stimulus for the emotional state in all its manifestations. In dealing with 'the chiefest' causes of 'accidental' melancholy, Burton lists '*Death of Friends*', 'Amongst which, loss and death of friends may challenge a first place, *multi tristantur . . .*'. But loss can also be temporary and still cause distress, and he asks rhetorically, 'If parting of friends, absence alone can work such violent effects, what shall death do, when they must eternally be separated, never in this world to meet again?'[6]

4. A Word: 'Adieu'

A single word denoting loss and 'goneness' is 'adieu', most famously associated with the Ghost in *Hamlet*, the play which is a recurrent reference point for Keats in his writing career. It occurs first in 'Lamia':

> 'It cannot be – Adieu!' So said, she rose
> Tip-toe with white arms spread. He, sick to lose
> The amorous promise of her lone complain . . .

It occurs no less than three times in 'Ode to a Nightingale':

> Adieu! the fancy cannot cheat so well
> As she is fam'd to do, deceiving elf.

Adieu! adieu! thy plaintive anthem fades
Past the near meadows, over the still stream,
Up the hill-side; and now 'tis buried deep
In the next valley-glades . . .

(ll. 71–8)

And finally in 'Ode on Melancholy':

She dwells with Beauty – Beauty that must die;
And Joy, whose hand is ever at his lips
Bidding adieu; and aching Pleasure nigh,
Turning to poison while the bee-mouth sips . . .

(ll. 21–4)

Although the word itself is not used in 'To Autumn', yet the swallows gathering to migrate in the last line are effectively saying *'au revoir'* if not 'adieu' to the post-harvest landscape, preparing to migrate until they return in spring. Like the ambivalence of loss in most of the poems, the occurrences tend to qualify a fully negative sense of finality, since 'adieu' in each case marks a transitional experience, an arrested point between the past and future. Such a pattern of necessary relinquishment was deeply ingrained in Keats's thinking, recurring not only in poems but also in his famous allegories of life as a series of emotional changes, 'The vale of Soul-making' and 'a large Mansion of many Apartments'. In an earlier sonnet which is not in this volume but was published posthumously in 1838,[7] 'On Sitting Down to Read King Lear Once Again', the word 'adieu' had described Keats's poetic journey away from romance to realism, viewed as something equally lost and gained:

Adieu! for once again the fierce dispute,
Betwixt damnation and impassion'd clay
Must I burn through . . .

Significantly, this sonnet was composed while Keats was writing *Endymion*, which he regarded as – or at least hoped would prove – a transitional work from his immersion in romance to a more bracing engagement with painful reality.

What joins the theme of loss and the word 'adieu' is another general pattern which runs through *1820* as an attempt to evade loss through a repeated enterprise of peering into past time and retrieving it for the present. The process is the topic of a recent book by William A. Ulmer, *John Keats: Reimagining History*.[8] This theme of the passing of time is, Ulmer argues, a feature of Keats's poetry throughout his career, but I will argue more particularly that it is a defining thematic feature of the 1820 volume. Each occurrence is not a simple repetition but a set of variations.

The past as irretrievable is especially insistent in the romances and odes: 'no sooner said, | Than with a frightful scream she vanished' ('Lamia'); 'To-day thou wilt not see him, nor to-morrow, | And the next day will be a day of sorrow' ('Isabella' XXIX); 'And they are gone: ay, ages long ago . . .' ('Eve of St. Agnes'); 'Fled is that music' ('Ode to a Nightingale'), 'not a soul to tell | Why thou art desolate, can e'er return' ('Ode on a Grecian Urn'). In the shorter, more comic poems, the historical past of Elizabethan poets is recaptured, while seizing the time before it passes is central to 'Ode on Melancholy'. The passing of time underpins the sequential perceptions in 'To Autumn', and here there is an implied undertone of reference to cyclicity and future repetition, qualifying an apparently gentle dismissal of each aspect of the season in turn. As in 'On Melancholy', there is a concentration on the present as sufficient in itself without thought for the future: 'Where are the songs of Spring? Ay, where are they? | Think not of them, thou hast thy music too'. Time is such a ubiquitous concern in Keats's poetry that it will recur, but at this stage it is enough to mention it as another thread running through the 1820 volume and binding the poems together.

5. A Poetic Reference: Milton's 'L'Allegro' and 'Il Penseroso'.

Behind the antitheses presented in these poems hovers a literary reference familiar to Keats, Milton's 'L'Allegro' and 'Il Penseroso', a pair of poems obviously intended to be read together as a single work extolling the respective virtues of two apparently opposed states of poetic inspiration. The eighteenth-century poet and critic Thomas Warton (an editor of Milton's works who himself wrote poetry on melancholy) had suggested that Milton's poems in turn were inspired by a poem subtitled 'A Dialogue between Pleasure and Pain', prefixed to Burton's *Anatomy of Melancholy*.[9] The first of Milton's poems is based on 'mirth' and pastoral nature, and the second on contemplative seriousness and scholarly 'divinest melancholy' in its most benign early modern sense, a 'sage and holy' state. Since the domain of Mirth or 'l'Allegro' is daylight and that of Melancholy or 'Il Penseroso' is twilight and the darkness of night, the obvious intention is to suggest they are not in fact incompatible but complementary and equally necessary states in human experience. The lighter poems grouped together in Keats's collection ('Fancy', 'Bards of Passion and of Mirth', 'Lines on the Mermaid Tavern' and 'Robin Hood') are written in the same form and rhyming couplets as Milton's,[10] and in a similar spirit, and many of the lines in Milton must have proved irresistible inspiration for the younger writer of *Poems* (1817) and *Endymion*: 'Such sights as youthful Poets dream | On summer eves by haunted stream'. Scholarly editors such as Miriam Allott and John Barnard cite Milton's work as a direct source for 'Welcome joy and welcome sorrow', a short poem probably written in October 1818, which it seems Keats considered for inclusion in *1820*.

The literary reference has a wider significance for the volume. Most of the antitheses identified above turn on poles of 'joy' and 'sorrow' and on Milton's twin states. In the earlier poems such as 'Lamia' and 'Isabella' they are strongly opposed and seen as incompatible, with different forms of melancholy (in the case of 'Lamia', intellectual 'thoughtfulness', in 'Isabella' love melancholy and grief) dismayingly destroying the early mirth of love. In the middle of the volume, and most tellingly in 'Nightingale' and 'Grecian Urn', the two are held in opposed suspension, and as in Milton's poems they are regarded as separate and temporally incompatible perspectives, so that we can have only one at a time. Towards the end of the collection, however, we find the kind of inclusive vision clearly intended by Milton in linking his two poems, and by Keats in 'Welcome joy and welcome sorrow'. In 'To Autumn' and 'Ode on Melancholy' opposing emotions complement each other as a comprehensive view of life and poetry. It is this direction, from antithesis to synthesis, which I suggest forms a narrative direction in *1820* as a whole, as one of the 'dozen features of Propriety' in the volume. Moreover, there are touches throughout which seem intertextually associated with Milton's duality. 'L'Allegro' begins by banishing 'loathed Melancholy' which is consigned to places of 'brooding darkness' and replaced by 'heart-easing Mirth' defined as joy in nature, and innocent love. It bears comparison with the opening of 'Ode to a Nightingale', where a spirit of heartache and 'drowsy numbness' gives way to the 'beechen green' of summer and 'full-throated ease' of the nightingale's song. In 'Il Penseroso' the nightingale is hailed as 'Sweet bird that shunn'st the noise of folly, | Most musical, most Melancholy', singing the song of Philomel, 'In her sweetest, saddest plight', and the pair of poems in Milton's collection are followed by his sonnet addressed to the Nightingale. 'Il Penseroso' also begins by banishing the converse state, now positioned as frivolous: 'Hence, vain deluding joyes' and idle pleasure and the sleepiness of 'fickle Pensioners of *Morpheus* train' which bears comparison with Keats's 'some dull opiate' which 'Lethewards had sunk', and more generally with the opening dismissal of different forms of mirth in the 'Nightingale' ode. As a corollary, 'Ode on Melancholy' reinterprets the more destructive and sinister melancholy mood as one that is positive, life-affirming and creative. The strategy of defining a mood by challenging its opposite runs through other Keatsian lines, such as 'No, no, go not to Lethe . . .' ('Ode on Melancholy'), and 'Heard melodies are sweet, but those unheard I Are sweeter' ('Ode on a Grecian Urn'). Foregoing one state to achieve an initially incompatible opposite may seem in theory necessary, but in the implied composite view that is surely Milton's longer purpose in juxtaposing 'L'Allegro' with 'Il Penseroso', and the spirit which prevails throughout Keats's collection, it seems that a fusion of both are possible in poetry – 'Welcome joy and welcome sorrow'. By reading *1820* in the light of Milton's 'L'Allegro' and 'Il Penseroso', we begin to glimpse a kind of overarching perspective in the collection as a whole, and one which will be the subject in the rest of this book.

6. Antithetical States

Enchantment and disenchantment, and the model of 'L'Allegro' and 'Il Penseroso' are examples of conceptual antithesis in *1820* but there are others, suggesting a more general pattern running through the collection. Opposing states recall Keats's words in his late letter from Rome to Brown (30 November, 1820) in which he writes about 'the knowledge of contrast, feeling for light and shade, all that information (primitive sense) necessary for a poem . . .'.[11] In the three romances the antitheses are bold and clear and help structure the stories. In 'Lamia' there are a set of very obvious contrasts. The apparently beautiful young woman is in reality a serpent, and her disguise is penetrated and destroyed by the 'sophist': 'do not all charms fly I At the mere touch of philosophy?'. At the same time her love for Lycius is genuine and at odds with her hidden, duplicitous nature; and even as snake her appearance has a dazzling, peacock-like beauty of its own, enhanced by the poetry: 'Vermilion-spotted, golden, green, and blue'. In 'Isabella' the major contrast is the moral one between the rapacious, commercially motivated brothers, and the young lovers, and it is mirrored in terms of place, between the repressive, courtly domicile and the forest. In 'The Eve of St Agnes' the various contrasts are imaged as settings and objects which have human and emotional analogues: sounds of drunken carousing contrast with silent corridors and the hushed bedroom, darkness with vibrant colours, the outer chill with the warmth of Madeline's clothes. Even objects can be both material and immaterial, inert and yet mysteriously volitional, such as carpets lifted by the wind, and take on a curious inner life of their own. There is an overarching set of contrasts between the unruly social world and the privacy and inwardness of Madeline's distraction, opening out into the world of wind and rain when the lovers flee. More contentious is the status of Porphyro himself, who has been seen as a liberator or violator, as though embodying a moral antithesis.[12]

The rest of the works in the collection are separated in the text (but not the table of contents) by the subtitle 'and other poems', and although they are manifestly different in tone and brevity from the narrative poems, they too are built on internal antitheses between the past and present status of poets and poetry. 'Fancy', 'Ode' ('Bards of Passion and of Mirth'), 'Lines on the Mermaid Tavern' and 'Robin Hood' all negotiate between on the one hand, pleasure, poetry and the past; and on the other, the banalities of diurnal existence. In 'Ode to a Nightingale', music gives way to silence, ecstatic vision is disrupted by 'waking dream' into reality, death consciousness floods at the instant of most vibrant imaginative life and intensity. In 'Ode on a Grecian Urn' the permanence of art is drawn into stark contrast with ephemeral and changing circumstances of life. These two odes, alongside 'Ode to Psyche', consciously turn on contrast between a realm of the creative imagination standing apart from reality but blurring the margins and allowing the two to intersect. 'To Autumn' and 'Ode on Melancholy' incorporate and sublimate many of the contrasts presented in the other works. An unsung narrative of the collection steers us from mutually exclusive polarities, such as 'Love in a hut, with water and a crust, | Is – Love forgive us! – cinders, ashes dust . . .' ('Lamia'), towards inclusivity of vision and the dissolving of antithetical states into complex, often paradoxical forms of unified experience.

7. Dialectic and Paradox

Another way of approaching the antitheses running through the collection is to suggest that contradictions are set up as debating positions around common themes, posing opposites in order to reconcile them in some way, often using paradoxical thinking. This might be illustrated by comparing the duality set up in the first poem, 'Lamia', with 'Ode on Melancholy', arguably the last if we do not consider 'Hyperion' to be Keats's intended closure. One way of explaining this is to focus on an apparently 'half-random' detail – eyesight – which occurs in the former as a problem and in the latter as a solution. This may not have been conscious in Keats's mind, but it constitutes another of the multiple ways in which the poet's imagination is working with a unified vision resolving underlying problems through the volume.

In 'Lamia' the eyes are mentioned in significant contexts, both in terms of their own visual power to entrance, and as acuity of sight, the ability to penetrate surfaces and see depths. In some versions of the story the lamia was distinguished by her eyes, which were removable. This is not mentioned by Keats, but he does mention eyes no fewer than thirty-four times in the poem, with a range of related applications, so they are certainly significant. Lamia as serpent is described as having 'eyes like a peacock' (presumably referring to the 'eyes' on the bird's parti-coloured tail rather than the imperious but beady eyes). Her eyes are amongst the most potently expressive evidence of her conflicted feelings: 'And for her eyes: what could such eyes do there I But weep, and weep, that they were born so fair'. The serpent's eyes are later described as 'melancholy'. When transformed into a woman she veils herself and avoids company in order to forestall 'the love-glances of unlovely eyes' of others. Her own eyes bloom, 'like new flowers at morning song of bees' giving up their honey. In the form of a snake her eyes are revealing of her state, more demonic this time:

> Her eyes in torture fix'd, and anguish drear,
> Hot, glaz'd, and wide, with lid-lashes all sear,
> Flash'd phosphor and sharp sparks, without one cooling tear.

When she sees Lycius it is her eyes which are the first agency of love, and mutually 'soon his eyes had drunk her beauty up' when she appears as a woman. However, when the philosopher enters the banquet he is identified as sharp-eyed, 'with eye severe', and unflinching in his ocular attention:

> The bald-head philosopher
> Had fix'd his eye, without a twinkle or stir
> Full on the alarmed beauty of the bride,
> Brow-beating her fair form, and troubling her sweet pride.

'Begone, foul dream!' he cries, and she responds in alarm, 'Shut, shut those juggling eyes, thou ruthless man!'. In Lycius's view, the sophist's 'lashless eyelids stretch I Around his demon eyes! ... My sweet bride withers at their potency'. However, the relentlessly clear-sighted 'eyes still I Relented not, nor mov'd'. Throughout 'Lamia', then, eyes are especially ambiguous but powerful in their operation. They can dazzle, they can create love, but also they can deceive. They can demystify illusions and reveal concealed truth by penetrating disguises and appearances. Even when piercingly observant of reality there is something dismaying and cold-hearted about the process, since philosophy – or science – is said by the equivocating narrator to 'Unweave a rainbow, as it erewhile made I The tender-person'd Lamia melt into a shade', revealing the vulnerability of the loving feelings of her identity beneath the appearance. The contradictions are not (and need not be) resolved within 'Lamia', since their ambiguities are purposeful in the poem's design, but they focus a problematical set of relationships between love and reality, beauty and truth, which runs through the poem and more generally troubled Keats. What we see may not be 'truth'.

By the end of the collection, however, in 'Ode on Melancholy', we find a possible resolution of this troubling dichotomy of eyesight, albeit one that is succinctly expressed in the shorter lyric poem. Whereas ambivalence had prevailed in 'Lamia', here a preference and even a commitment is made, with a marked difference of attitude focusing on appearances:

> Then glut thy sorrow on a morning rose,
> Or on the rainbow of the salt sand-wave,
> Or on the wealth of globed peonies;
> Or if thy mistress some rich anger shows,
> Emprison her soft hand, and let her rave,
> And feed deep, deep upon her peerless eyes.

The ode proclaims that the eyes have their own self-consistent power which offers a choice to a lover of what to believe, since their effect need not be feared but instead can be accepted and embraced in the moment before it disappears. The ode implicitly concludes that, like transient flowers and rainbows, a lover's eyes are not appropriate targets for the destructive scientist's analytical mind, but instead can be simply enjoyed in the richness of a moment before it passes. Only those who can accept and be willingly beguiled are allowed a glimpse of the fatal but fascinating 'temple of Delight', '*seen* of none save him whose strenuous tongue I Can burst Joy's grape against his palate fine' (my italics). In a state of such intensity the contradictions between love and knowledge dissolve, so that the debate set up in 'Lamia' is at least avoided and perhaps resolved. Even if the poet knows only too well the power of the eyes to delude or to destroy, he advocates giving free rein to enjoy the sensory and emotional richness of a fully apprehended present instance, in order to undergo an unrepeatable experience of ecstatic melancholy, which otherwise we would be the poorer to have missed. By implication, the same can be said of the potential lies and seductive delights of poetry, a preoccupation of both Spenser and Milton, the poets most influential on Keats alongside Shakespeare. 'Ode on Melancholy', especially coming immediately after the air of calm acceptance expressed in 'To Autumn' (which is full of 'seeing' in a different spirit), can be read as subverting an oversharp dichotomy between knowledge gained through either the senses or the ratiocinative mind; imagination or reason.

I have never yet been able to perceive how any thing can be known for truth by consequitive reasoning – and yet it must be – Can it be that even the greatest Philosopher ever arrived at his goal without putting aside numerous objections – However, it may be, O for a Life of Sensations rather than of Thoughts![13]

The volume as a whole moves towards a point of believing that beauty and truth need not be at war, as they are in 'Lamia'.

8. Beauty and Truth

The enigmatic collocation of beauty and truth is not confined to 'Ode on a Grecian Urn' where the phrase is explicitly used, for it occurs in some form in perhaps all the poems in the volume. Ever since Plato linked the two, initially in the *Phaedrus* and *The Symposium*, writers and philosophers have debated terms in tandem. William A. Ulmer provides a category of usages in which the linked words were a Regency commonplace, especially in Keats's cultural *milieu* comprising such artists as Haydon and Hazlitt.[14] Here we are on well-trodden Keatsian ground. In 'Lamia' the concepts are presented as an exclusive choice – beauty *or* truth – with the implication that they may not, perhaps even cannot coexist. By the time we come to 'To Autumn' and 'Ode on Melancholy' the two are presented as indissolubly linked as one, since beauty *is* truth in the intensity of the moment, should we choose to see it this way. As Keats put it in an early letter, 'the excellence of every Art is its intensity, capable of making all disagreeables evaporate, from their being in close relationship with Beauty & Truth'.[15] Keats's thinking on beauty and truth, I have argued elsewhere, was influenced also by Shakespeare's Sonnets. The exact phrase is used in Sonnets 14 ('I read such art I As truth and beauty shall together thrive'), 101 ('Both truth and beauty on my love depends') and in two lines in 54 ('By how much more doth beauty beauteous seem I By that sweet ornament that truth doth give!'). The respective juxtapositioning and merging of beauty and truth is so conspicuous that it seems to be one of Keats's conscious preoccupations in the volume, rather than occurring 'half at Random'.

By looking at the different ways of understanding possible relationships between beauty and truth, we can see reasons why 'Nightingale', 'Grecian Urn' and 'Psyche' occupy a literally central place, and why they are in this order. Before these three, the romances propose that beauty and truth may be in opposition, depending on how we define 'truth' in each case. 'Lamia' is the most schematic, since the beautiful appearance of the woman is not consistent with the truth of her serpentine being nor with her immortality, and the dénouement uncovers the discrepancy through the eyes of the truth-telling philosopher: beauty is *not* truth but deception, and nor is truth beautiful. In 'The Eve of St Agnes' truth is a more negotiable quality depending on the reader's perspective, but it is still at least part of a conceptual opposition. On the one hand, we are presented with truth as unpleasant reality, the brutal and sordid family environment trapping Madeline and the factual existence of death at the end of the poem. These contrast with the more idealised and youthful lovers who finally escape, aligned as they are with images of beauty and with a different kind of truth, to the emotions if not practical reality. 'Isabella', just as clearly as 'Lamia', turns on one opposition between love and an unsympathetic, materialistic family context represented by the acquisitive and resentful brothers, and another when the lovers are separated by Lorenzo's death, substituting a kind of morbid fetishisation which takes over Isabella's grief-stricken feelings. In all three narrative poems, and in different ways in each, resolution of beauty and truth seems not to be on offer, as though they pose a fundamental problem of moral categories which will be explored more philosophically in the succeeding poems.

The first three odes bring the terms into the open as a dialectic, leading to paradoxes rather than a simple opposition. Once again, these will be discussed in more detail later in relation to melancholy, but for now the bare bones can be summarised in a way that may suggest why Keats placed them in the order in which they appear rather than necessarily in the order of composition. 'Ode to a Nightingale' presents as 'truth' the beauty of sound, whether of a nocturnal birdsong or music more generally, in the particular sense of its ability to transform the listener's emotional state in a temporal sense, suspending in an all-encompassing fashion reference to anything outside the sound. It creates a whole imaginative landscape and mental model of all-inclusive reality, in an ecstatic state which verges on the oblivion and annihilation of death: 'Now more than ever seems it rich to die'. Paradoxically, sound exists only in time, with a beginning and end, yet at its most harmonically and melodically intense it can create an apprehension of timelessness which obliterates all thought of 'before and after'. Once it starts and until it stops, beautiful music seems to exist in its own state of suspended ever-presence, without past or future. While it operates, it offers a beauty which holds its own alternative truth. The analogy with the word-music of poetry is inescapable. But when the music stops, the listener is returned to the mundane reality which prevailed before it started, as a kind of unavoidable bedrock of a more diurnal kind of truth that cannot be evaded forever, except in death. As in 'Lamia' this truth is not beautiful but sobering and even dismaying, and casts doubt on the previous experience as either 'a vision or waking dream' which, however truthful and beautiful, cannot be sustained.

In 'Ode on a Grecian Urn' the dialectic is shifted to an art form that conversely exists only outside time, static pictorial representation which excludes sequential time altogether. This too can be self-evidently 'true' but in a quite different sense, existing as that which cannot change and is untouched by the vicissitudes of external reality. The beauty of this kind of art is self-sufficient and does not depend on the viewer's feelings, though the stasis of the artistic representation can, in a limited temporal zone, invite construction of a hypothetical narrative around the events depicted. Its truth is on its own uncompromising and unchanging terms, not the perceiver's, which is why it is the urn itself that delivers its own 'moral': '"Beauty is truth, truth beauty"'. However (at least in the version printed in *1820*), an exclusionary *coda* seems to be delivered by the poet: '– that is all | Ye know on earth, and all ye need to know'. This places the poet in an intermediary's position, able to understand and communicate the truth of art while equally existing in the viewer's time-bound reality, and in turn leads on to the next poem, 'Ode to Psyche' where the poet adopts the stance of an artist creating the illusion of a truthful and beautiful but separate realm of mythology, where the goddess Psyche dwells. Here the poet as creator is the arbiter, 'I see, and sing, by my own eyes inspired | So let me be thy choir . . .'; 'Yes, I will be thy priest . . .'. It is the poet as imaginative artist who can bridge the realms of beauty in art and the reality in which people live, bringing the absolute truth of the former into the relative element of the latter, making beauty into truth for the reader.

The next poem, 'Fancy' ('Ever let the fancy roam'), speaks from inside poetry's pleasure-dwelling vision, presented almost as a free-floating abstraction without need for an intermediary poet. 'Fancy' speaks for itself as the central, expressive consciousness. The following couple, 'Ode' ('Bards of Passion and of Mirth') and 'Lines on the Mermaid Tavern' ('Souls of Poets dead and gone'), generalise further by arguing that dead poets have two beings, one in the past when they were alive and the other incorporating their works which post-date their lives and continue to have a posthumous existence in terms of their beauty and truth. Taken together, then, the sequence of poems presents a kind of narrative development proceeding at first dialectically and increasingly synthesising, the problematical and teasing relationship between truth and beauty. It is a recurrent reference point which was insistently a part of Keats's thinking when he wrote and collected the poems, as one of the more conscious among the 'dozen features of Propriety' that could bind the collection together, and another pattern weaving through the sequence of poems in *1820*.

9. Associational Imagery

The sets of internal cohesion or multidimensional unity suggested so far have dwelt on thematic concerns or an implied, unfolding – if oscillating – narrative, but there are other kinds of logic stitching the works together. One is the apparently adventitious ('half at Random') sequential process of 'one thing follows another', driven by association of ideas and words rather than by reason and narrative direction. Since the poems had been composed at different times, the links between each are unlikely to have been part of any prior, preconceived plan, but occur when the poet collects and places the poems in a certain order for publication. Inevitably, however, Keats was obviously thinking intensely about certain preoccupations when he was writing the poems in a relatively short span of time, most during early 1819, so it is not surprising that there are intrinsic links. One would expect the poems to 'rub off on each other', and also that later, with hindsight, they could be arranged to look as though one thought process helped to generate the next. This principle of associational, apparently organic growth was what struck Keats about the writing of his 'presider', Shakespeare, especially within and between Sonnets:

> I neer found so many beauties in the sonnets – they seem to be full of fine things said unintentionally – in the intensity of working out conceits – Is this to be borne? Hark ye!
>   'When lofty trees I see barren of leaves
>   Which [erst] From heat did canopy the he[a]rd,
>   And Summer's green all girded up in sheaves,
>   Borne on the bier with white and bristly beard.'[16]

The quotation from Shakespeare's Sonnet 12 offers a variation on the 'dozen features of Propriety' passage in the way it conceives of poetic creation as partly a matter of luck ('unintentionally') and partly of internally coherent thought: 'fine things said unintentionally – in the intensity of working out conceits –'. Even this brilliant, throw-away statement by Keats casually demonstrates its own inner verbal associativeness in its chime between 'unintentionally' and 'intensity', oddly paralleling the fusing of 'half at Random' and unexpected 'Propriety'. The idea implies that Shakespeare sustained the momentum by associative image-making, rather than by conscious forward planning. Keats admiringly dubs him 'the whim King!', a wonderfully lucky phrase which captures the apparently arbitrary but 'whimsically' fortuitous way Shakespeare thinks through progressions of related images, giving the impression of not knowing where they will lead as he writes. In his own 'unintentional' way Keats has identified and linked a characteristic of many of Shakespeare's sonnets, where the poem starts with an image which, by either word, sound, or sense association, leads on to the next image. In the sonnet he quotes, for example, we can trace the progression of thought developed associationally through linkages between pictorial images which goes something like this: trees > without leaves > thus depriving cattle of shelter > post-harvest > sheaves of corn > carried on a 'bier' with its funereal association > old age > death. There is an added level in the implicit but unstated equation of 'sheaves' of corn with pages of a writer's book, bound in 'sheaves' and outliving the author, tying in the organic processes of nature with the creation of a poem or volume. In this sense, although Keats was not to know it, his 1820 volume was to be his own 'Summer's green all girded up in sheaves'. That he himself internalised Shakespeare's method is most amply shown in 'To Autumn'.

10. Links from Poem to Poem

We might pursue this particular point about Shakespeare's style a little further, since we notice links not only within but also between some of the sonnets, and although we have no way of knowing whether the order of publication was authorised by Shakespeare (nor even if it is a consciously ordered collection at all), it seems undeniable that some sonnets 'answer' their predecessor, as though each is giving birth to the next. For example, Sonnet 23 ends with the image of 'eyes' which in turn opens 24; 33 ends on the image of the sun clouded which opens 34; 46 ends with imagery of eye and heart which exactly mirrors the start of 47; and so on. 57–8 (slave), 71–2 (after my death), 111–12 (pity), 113–14 (mind), 98–9 (poison and remedies), 131–2 (black), 135–6 (play on the name of 'Will'), 140–1 (eyes). The two final sonnets (153 and 154) are obviously presented as a pair. 97 to 99 can be read as tracing the seasons ('How like a winter . . .', 'From you I have been absent in the spring', and summer flowers). In the case of Keats's collection, we can find similar linkages through words and associations – perhaps not so much between the three longer poems, but the shorter ones show signs of being arranged to lead on from each to the next by a connection probably noticed only 'afterwards' when 'confirmed by [the poet's] judgment'. Cessation of music and a question close 'Ode to a Nightingale' ('Fled is that music: – Do I wake or sleep?') while 'Ode on a Grecian

Urn', as though in answer, begins with 'unheard melodies', and the first stanza ends with questions paralleling the interrogative conclusion to 'Nightingale': 'What pipes and timbrels? What wild ecstasy?'. Next, 'Ode on a Grecian Urn' ends with the image 'With forest branches and the trodden weed' and 'Ode to Psyche' opens with 'I wander'd in a forest thoughtlessly'. In turn, 'Psyche' ends with 'all the gardener Fancy e'er could feign' and 'Fancy' itself comes next, its first line being 'Ever let the Fancy roam'. This poem is about poetry and is followed by one about poets: 'Bards of Passion and of Mirth . . . | Ye have souls in heaven too, | Double-lived in regions new'. The bards living in two worlds spill over into 'Lines on the Mermaid Tavern' – Souls of Poets dead and gone, | What Elysium have ye known'. This poem ends with another rhetorical question, 'What Elysium have ye known . . . | Choicer than the Mermaid Tavern?', which seems immediately to be forcefully answered in the negative in 'Robin Hood: 'No! those days are gone away'. In turn, the refrain of 'Robin Hood' ('Gone . . . ', 'Dead and gone') is gently answered in 'To Autumn', with another refutation, in at least the opening vision of things held in a process of 'maturing' apparently without end, and bees which 'think warm days will never cease'. The next verse is presented as the suspended animation of pictorial art, and the next reintroduces movement and change. 'To Autumn' leads us to the brink of death again in the final verse (at least in 'the soft-dying day' and the incipient end of the season), but this is followed by 'Ode on Melancholy' which syntactically pulls us back from the temporal ledge: 'No, no, go not to Lethe . . . ', though it ends with a kind of fulfilled death and final destiny. Some of these suggested links may seem slight and stretched, but taken together they suggest a poet who is presenting an ordering of his poems through exercising 'judgment', highlighting links which suggest 'fine things said unintentionally – in the intensity of working out conceits . . .'. Some examples follow in the next section.

11. 'Stitching' Imagery

A related way in which poems in the 1820 anthology are knitted together lies in more pervasive imagery which recurs from poem to poem across the collection. Many examples are detailed elsewhere in this book or already identified by Fraistat and editors, and here I intend to stick to a particular line of thought in attempting to answer one puzzling question. The first poem in any collection may have a special, privileged position in relation to the rest that follow, since in some ways it is a bellwether, offering a clue to what is to follow. Keats and his publishers at one stage considered starting with 'The Eve of St Agnes',[17] which most modern readers find the most satisfying and perhaps the most accessible of the romances, but they finally decided to begin with 'Lamia'. Why? Keats's own answers seem to have included his thought that this poem was arresting, having 'that sort of fire in it which must take hold of people in some way',[18] but other suggestions might occur to us. One possible answer is briefly mentioned above, that the first three poems, although all influenced by the Romantic Gothic revival, depict stories told in three consecutive chronological periods. 'Lamia' is set in Cretan antiquity, while 'Isabella' is a retelling of Boccaccio's 'old tale' in the *Decameron*, set in a late medieval period edging into the emergent capitalism of the early modern period through the brothers' commercialism built upon slave labour. The temporal setting of 'The Eve of St Agnes' is more indeterminate, though with its conspicuous influence from *Romeo and Juliet* and its rich architectural detail, it seems placed in the high Renaissance. (This may itself be another piece of evidence for the anomaly of 'Hyperion' at the end, since the latter breaks chronology by returning to the world of classical gods.) In the 'Other Poems' which follow the romances the poet speaks in the present tense, despite their recollective invocations of older times, while 'To Autumn' and 'Melancholy' are placed in an immediate, changing present tense.

In poetic style and genre the groups of poems are also different: 'Lamia' with its simple couplets in extended narrative, 'Isabella' in the Italianate *ottavo rima* befitting Boccaccio, 'The Eve of St Agnes' in Spenserian stanzas befitting its possible Elizabethan period – as Ian Jack summarises, the world of *The Faerie Queene*, *Romeo and Juliet*, Milton's minor poems, Browne's *Britannia's Pastorals*, Burton's *Anatomy of Melancholy* and others.[19] 'Ode to Psyche' and the more experimental, varied, and occasional odes and song-like *rondeaux* (so called by Keats though they are not quite in the conventional form of that genre) that follow, place attention on the presence of a shaping poet rather than the tale he tells. Jeffrey N. Cox reinforces the suggestion that the order implies an historical development of poetry, summarising thus:

> Read in the volume's sequence, the poems also offer, as Stuart Curran points out, an experiment with the modes of 'Greek (in couplets), Italian (in ottavo rima), and British (in Spenserian stanzas)' romance, as Keats plots a cultural movement from the classical past through the Christian middle ages to the present.[20]

Another reason for placing 'Lamia' first might be that it introduces explicitly most of the thematic concerns that occur later. Some of these have already been mentioned – beauty and truth, enchantment and disenchantment (Fraistat), the potential deceitfulness of fancy and imagination, problematical love, and so on. In addition, 'Lamia' anticipates a significant amount of the imagery that will recur in later poems. It can be seen to lead us into the whole, imaginative world of *1820* at its most resonantly detailed and embroidered level. This is another aspect which might have been more evident to the poet looking back as a reader and as *de facto* editor, exercising more critical 'judgment' than when he was writing individual poems 'half at Random' at different times, stimulated by specific and fluctuating circumstances without yet contemplating a completed anthology.

Other anticipations are initiated in 'Lamia' and recur in later poems. The image of budding flowers, for example, is presented in association with female sexuality in 'Lamia' – 'self-folding like a flower | That faints into itself at evening hour' – which is next attached to Madeline in 'Eve': 'As though a rose should shut, and be a bud again'. Later it is more generally indicative of fruitful nature, like the 'unseen' but aromatic landscape in 'Nightingale', and the process of buds turning into flowers in 'Psyche':

> With buds, and bells, and stars without a name,
> With all the gardener Fancy e'er could feign,
> Who, breeding flowers, will never breed the same.

In 'Fancy' we find 'And the enjoying of the spring | Fades as does its blossoming', and 'All the buds and bells of May'; and most memorably in 'To Autumn', 'to set budding more, | And still more, later flowers for the bees . . . '. Budding flowers are set up in 'Lamia' as a nightly occurrence, in 'Eve' as a once and forever turning point from innocence to experience, and in later poems captured as a potentially unending organic process, mirroring something of the collection's overall direction.

Another image, wine, flows freely in 'Lamia': 'merry wine, sweet wine' leads quickly to general jollity and inebriation; in 'Eve' the guests are 'Drown'd all in Rhenish and the sleepy mead'; 'O, for a draught of vintage' is the subject of the second verse of 'Nightingale', and 'Canary wine' as 'beverage divine' is served in the Mermaid Tavern. In 'Fancy', 'She will mix these pleasures up | Like three fit wines in a cup, | And thou shalt quaff it'; 'spicy ale' is also quaffed in 'Robin Hood'; while finally 'Veil'd melancholy' is seen of none 'save him whose strenuous tongue | Can burst Joy's grape against his palate fine'.

There are also feasts in 'Lamia': 'feasts and rioting', an 'Adonian feast' of fresh 'amorous herbs and flowers, newly reap'd', an aborted 'marriage feast and nuptial mirth', featuring tables laden with delicacies which later lie 'untasted'. In 'Eve' there are two feasts, the one an unruly public one hosted by the Baron which degenerates into a drunken cacophony, and the other private, intimate and lavish, prepared by Porphyro for Madeline, with 'lustrous salvers' gleaming in the moonlight. It is provided more to enhance the sensuous eroticism of the scene than as sustenance:

> And still she slept an azure-lidded sleep,
> In blanched linen, smooth, and lavender'd,
> While he from forth the closet brought a heap
> Of candied apple, quince, and plum, and gourd
> With jellies soother than the creamy curd,
> And lucent syrops, tinct with cinnamon;
> Manna and dates, in argosy transferr'd
> From Fez; and spiced dainties, every one,
> From silken Samarcand to cedar'd Lebanon.
> xxxi.
> These delicates he heap'd with glowing hand
> On golden dishes and in baskets bright
> Of wreathed silver: sumptuous they stand
> In the retired quiet of the night,
> Filling the chilly room with perfume light. –

Its function is presumably not to be consumed but to contribute purely to an exotic atmosphere, full of promise of a glamorous world elsewhere. Among the various rituals associated with St. Agnes Eve, food does feature, in the rather less appetising, stodgy sounding 'dumb cake' made by four people at midnight and placed under the dreamer's pillow, the essential, spartan ingredients being flour, water, sugar and plenty of salt. Theories vary about the name, some suggesting that it had to be made with friends in silence, others that it derives from the word for 'doom' in its positive sense meaning 'destiny'. The lover will reputedly appear in a dream holding a glass of water or of beer. Porphyro's spread, by contrast, is a positive Middle Eastern *dégustation* menu. In 'Robin Hood' there is more solid English fare, 'dainty pies of venison' to eat – 'O generous food!'. Incense is mentioned, if only for its absence, in both 'Lamia' ('sepulchred, where no kindled incense burns') and 'Ode on a Grecian Urn' ('no incense sweet'). It wafts through 'Nightingale' ('Nor what soft incense hangs upon the boughs'), 'Psyche' ('thy incense sweet'), and metaphorically in 'Eve' ('like pious incense from a censer old'), stimulating the olfactory sense. All this may not be compelling evidence of poetic unity, since things like budding flowers, wine and incense were among Keats's favourite images, the latter recurring in *Endymion* and in both 'Hyperion' fragments, but their repetition in *1820* is collective evidence of the Keatsian poetic landscape, and in each case it is notable that 'Lamia' initiates them, as though setting up an echoing chamber to operate in the rest. The poem does its job of opening the collection in the way Keats describes the internal connections in a letter: 'by merely pulling an apron string we set a pretty peal of Chimes at work – Let them chime on a while, with your patience, – '.[21] 'Lamia' pulls on the apron string and sets the 'Chimes at work' in the poems that follow.

12. Towards Melancholy

Among other images and linkages, there is one more item of significant 'Propriety' in opening the volume with 'Lamia' and closing with 'Ode on Melancholy'. At the end of the first poem Keats appends the one and only footnote in the book, quoting a passage from Robert Burton's *The Anatomy of Melancholy* as the source of the story. In some ways this is unnecessary, at least in the length of the quotation, since the narrative is clear enough in Keats's telling, and not all that closely tied to Burton's account. The reference to Burton is also quite obtrusive as the only footnote in the book, as though Keats has some larger acknowledgment in mind, to a 'presider' over the volume as a whole. The importance of Burton's book for Keats himself is spelt out in Chapter 5, and its significance for *1820* will, I hope, emerge in Chapter 6 as a pervading presence behind Keats's selection of poems, as his own poetic equivalent of an 'anatomy of melancholy' moving towards the celebratory assertion of 'Ode on Melancholy'. To the cultural and literary significance of this condition we now turn.

Notes

1. To Haydon, 10–11 May 1817, *LJK*, 1, p. 142.
2. To George and Georgiana Keats, 15–30 Apr., 1819, *LJK*, 2, pp. 105–6.
3. To Taylor, 27 Feb. 1818, *LJK*, 1, p. 238.
4. Jack Stillinger, 'Keats's extempore effusions: Questions of intentionality', pp. 307–20, 309.
5. Fraistat, *The Poem and the Book*, p. 126.
6. Robert Burton, Book 1, First Section, Memb. IV, Subsect. VII.
7. *Plymouth and Devenport Weekly*, 8 November 1838; transcribed by Keats in his Folio edition of Shakespeare's works.
8. Ulmer, *John Keats: Reimagining History*.
9. Warton, p. 94 fn. For more on Warton, see ch. 4.
10. Barnard, *John Keats: 21st-Century Oxford Authors*, p. 620 fn.
11. To Brown, 30 November, 1820, *LJK*, 2, p. 360.
12. See Jack Stillinger, *Reading the Eve of St Agnes: The Multiples of Complex Literary Transaction*.

13. To Bailey, 22 November 1817, *LJK*, 1, p. 185.
14. Ulmer, *John Keats: Reimagining History*, pp. 150–3.
15. To George and Tom Keats, 21 December 1817, *LJK*, 1, p. 192.
16. To Reynolds, 22 November, 1817 (quoting Sonnet 12), *LJK*, 1, p. 189.
17. Keats, *The Complete Poems* ed. Miriam Allott, p. 451; *KC*, 1, p. 105; Barnard, *21st Century Oxford Authors*, p. 610.
18. To the George Keatses, 18 September 1819, *LJK*, 2, p. 189.
19. Jack, p. 191.
20. Cox, '*Lamia, Isabella,* and *The Eve of St Agnes*: Eros and "Romance"', pp. 53–68, pp. 56–7; citing Stuart Curran, p. 150.
21. To Reynolds 3 May 1818, *LJK*, 1, p. 280.

Melancholy

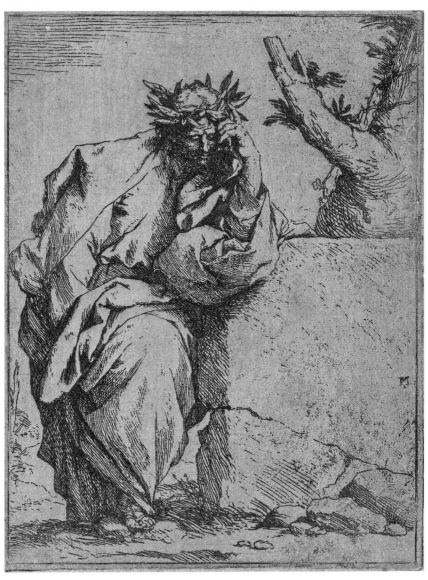

4.1 Jusepe Ribera's etching 'The Poet' (1620–1), Art Gallery of South Australia from the David Murray Bequest Fund 1949 (4910G183).

Chapter 4

Melancholy:
From Medical Condition to
Poetic Convention

In a literal sense, Keats's childhood years were spent under Melancholy since, as Nicholas Roe notes, opposite the Swan and Hoop inn and livery stables in Moorfields was Bedlam, presided over by Caius Cibber's twinned statues, 'Melancholy Madness' and 'Raving Madness'. Keats's retentive memory, Roe further suggests, carried this very image in his mind to re-emerge as the slumped and despondent fallen Titans in 'Hyperion'.[1] When he came to study medicine and walk the wards in Guy's Hospital, the indigent living embodiments of melancholy were to become all too real for him. But more than this, he had lived with the emotion throughout his life.

Keats was a connoisseur of melancholy in all its manifestations and reinventions, as it evolved from the ancient medical ailment down to his own day. It was a Renaissance 'Epidemical disease' (Robert Burton's phrase), and it developed into a Romantic-age poetic cult. The history of melancholy is vast and complex, and its intricacies have largely been lost in the modern, attenuated understanding of the word as 'pensive sadness'. However, the many conditions the word then described have been assimilated into modern psychology as a variety of mental disorders, so they have not disappeared altogether. Poetry too has played a preserving role, and it was a poet, Coleridge, who coined the word 'psychology' itself in English.[2] In this chapter, I present only the briefest of historical summaries to provide some context, preparing the way for more detailed inspection of Keats's markings and annotations on his copy of Robert Burton's *The Anatomy of Melancholy* in Chapter 5, followed by a melancholy-centred analysis of the individual poems in the 1820 collection in Chapter 6.

The word melancholy itself came originally from the Greek for 'black bile', one of the four humours making up the body of every person in the major paradigm of early medical theory associated with Hippocrates (*De Humoribus*) and Galen (*De Temperamentis*). These ideas had been

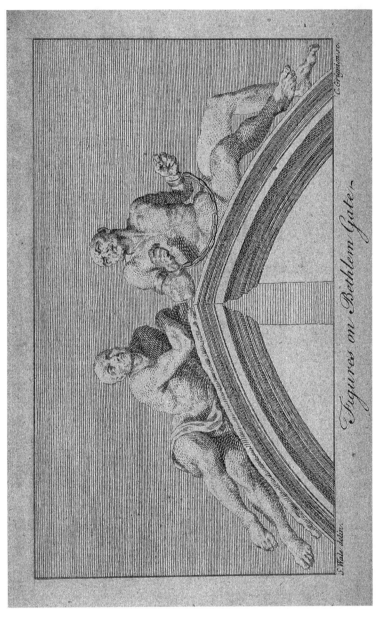

Figures on Bethlem Gates

4.2 Statues of 'melancholy' and 'raving' madness, each reclining on one half of a pediment, formerly crowning the gates at Bethlem (Bedlam) Hospital. Engraving by C. Grignion after S. Wale after C. Cibber, 1680. Credit: Wellcome Library Collection CC.BY, b1183482.

underpinned and given authority by Aristotle's natural philosophy in *De Animalibus*. Surviving into the Renaissance, melancholy became the subject of book-length studies in English, such as those by Thomas Elyot (*The Castel of Helthe*, 1534), Timothy Bright (*A Treatise of Melancholie*, 1586), Thomas Wright (*The Passions of the Minde in Generall*, 1630) and Robert Burton (*The Anatomy of Melancholy*, 1621 and sundry revised editions). For these writers and practitioners there was no necessary disjunction between medicine and philosophy, nor between body, soul and mind. 'The mind's inclination follows the body's temperature' was an encapsulation attributed to Galen. If the body was sick, then so most likely was the mind, and in more serious cases, the soul was also in trouble. When the humours were in balance then good health and a balanced temperament prevailed, but if the humours were 'dis-tempered' or unbalanced, then body and mind suffered equally, fields of study which we would differentiate as physiology and psychology. Burton succinctly lists the temperamental characteristics in his synoptic table of contents:

- Humours
  - Sanguine are merry still, laughing, pleasant, meditating on plays, women, music, &c.
  - Phlegmatic, slothful, dull, heavy, &c.
  - Choleric, furious, impatient, subject to hear and see strange apparitions, &c.
  - Black, solitary, sad; they think they are bewitched, dead, &c.
- Or mixed of these four humours adust, or not adust, infinitely varied.

'Infinitely varied' certainly encapsulates his own version of melancholy. The words are still in our vocabulary with broadly identical meanings, except for 'adust', meaning literally 'scorched, burnt black' from Latin and more metaphorically 'gloomy, melancholic'. Even the relatively cheerful sanguine type could evince alarming symptoms when excessive. Blood (hot and moist, affecting the heart) although normally promoting a 'pleasant' temperament, yet in excess could cause feverish physical and overexcitable mental conditions ('enthusiasm' had a pejorative edge, denoting religious obsessiveness). Fiery yellow bile (hot and dry, affecting the gall bladder) caused anger, choleric aggressiveness, envy and jealousy. Watery phlegm (cold and moist, associated with the brain) resulted in coughs, colds, general debility and a 'phlegmatic', lethargic temperament. All these could manifest in differing states of melancholy, but its specific province was when black bile came to predominate (cold and dry, affecting the spleen), with a catalogue of unfortunate emotional results, including potentially the even more dangerous condition of 'sadness' which might end in suicide.[3] Melancholy darkened the world in the mind of the sufferer, causing a huge range of pathological states including (at least in Burton's panoptic view) grief, hysteria, love-melancholy afflicting young women especially as 'green sickness', religious despair, suicidal thoughts, and states that we now call depression, anxiety, and even insanity. Burton casts his net far wider than his predecessors seeing melancholic subgroups in all the humours, and including states such as mania, frenzy and artistic genius that were conventionally distinguished as being acute conditions rather than, as was melancholy, a temperamental tendency which left untreated would become chronic and constitutional. Shakespeare evidently saw the connections between 'sadness' and 'frenzy', for in the Induction to *The Comedy of Errors* the Messenger informs Christopher Sly of the plan (my italics),

> to play a pleasant comedy,
> *For so your doctors hold it very meet,*
> Seeing too much sadness hath congealed your blood,
> *And melancholy is the nurse of frenzy.*
> Therefore they thought it good you hear a play
> And frame your mind to mirth and merriment . . .'.
>
> (Induction II, 125–32)

This neatly captures Burton's method of classification, distinguishing between symptom, cause and cure. The binding link between the different types was that they were generally 'accompanied by symptoms of apparently groundless fear and sorrow',[4] and it is these emotions of doom and gloom that were at the heart of the affliction.

Dreams were considered by Aristotle and later commentators as being especially useful in diagnosing which particular humour might be disordered, causing physical and mental imbalance. There are, of course, dreams, visions and 'waking dreams' throughout Keats's poetry, none so vivid and focused on melancholy as the sonnet 'A Dream, after reading Dante's Episode of Paolo and Francesca', with its 'second circle of sad hell', where

> lovers need not tell
> Their sorrows. Pale were the sweet lips I saw,
> Pale were the lips I kissed, and fair the form
> I floated with, about that melancholy storm.

The connection between dreams and creativity came from the assumption that dream images, which self-evidently did not exist in the material world, were considered to spring from the imagination without rational oversight or control. Poets and artists did not need to be dreaming to enter such a state. The physiological explanation offered was that the humoural overbalancing had dislodged one's reason, the faculty which normally controlled the imagination, resulting not only in 'safe' dreams but also in waking delusions and hallucinatory images (*phantasms*), which could, in inspired and gifted subjects, result in creativity. When the mind and passions were fully stretched in nonrational imaginings under the influence of melancholy, it could also be the driver for creativity in those said to be born under Saturn (the main god of melancholy, and a god-character of special significance in Keats's later 'Hyperion' project), especially in the arts and literature. Paradoxically, melancholy in its active form could cause ecstasy, and some physicians associated it with genius. Aristotle was reputed to have asked (though the source seems in fact to have been his student, Theophrastus), 'Why is it that all men who have become outstanding in philosophy, statesmanship, poetry or the arts are melancholic?'[5] As Dryden was later epigrammatically to quip in *Absalom and Achitophel* (1681), 'Great wits are to madness near allied | And thin partitions do their bounds divide'. A lingering variant of this provided one quasi-medical explanation for Keats's later illness, which he was predisposed to accept:

> The Doctor assures me that there is nothing the matter with me except nervous irritability and a general weakness of the whole system which has proceeded from my anxiety of mind of late years and the too great excitement of poetry.[6]

As well as explaining apparent opposites like agony and ecstasy, lassitude and creativity, melancholy could cover many other emotions along a spectrum from negative to positive, depending on what humours were involved. Joan Fitzpatrick quotes the herbalists of Burton's time, John Gerard and Nicholas Culpepper, as listing eight 'commixtures' of humours: 'chollerick–melancholy, melancholy–chollerick, melancholy–sanguine, sanguine–melancholy, sanguine–Flegmatick, Flegmatick–sanguine, Flegmatick–chollerick, chollerick–Flegmatick (Galen & Culpepper 1653, F5v)'.[7] The sheer variety of kinds, comparable to Polonius's amusing taxonomy of mixed literary genres in *Hamlet*, is especially important to Burton, whose *Anatomy* is kaleidoscopic and comprehensive in its range, as we shall see in Chapter 5. As the art historians Fritz Saxl and Erwin Panofsky have shown, alongside the published early modern treatises on melancholy as a medical condition, there was also a rich tradition of iconographical images and works of art depicting melancholia, most memorably those by Lucas Cranach the Elder (1532) and by Albrecht Dürer, whose hauntingly enigmatic engraving *Melencolia I* (1514) is famous.[8] Laurinda Dixon has traced the artistic representations through art history, from Dürer s engravings of the scholarly melancholic, Saint Jerome, through to the nineteenth century.[9] There has also been plenty of 'melancholy art' in the twentieth and twenty-first centuries, and though it is not these days commonly called by this name it is regarded as springing from psychologically defined states of mind.[10]

The diversity of possible melancholic conditions stemmed from the fact that a specific type could be activated by one's profession, gender or temperamental predisposition, and some people were more prone than others. Ben Jonson's 'humours comedy' supplies many such character-types, as does Shakespeare,[11] and among them there were religious zealots (Jonson's Zeal-of-the-land Busy in *Bartholomew Fair* and Shakespeare's Malvolio), scholars (Hamlet), lovers (Ophelia and again Hamlet), rootless travellers often known as 'malcontents' (Shakespeare's Jaques in *As You Like It*, as diagnosed by Rosalind, and the 'sad' entrepreneurial Antonio in *The Merchant of Venice* who was possibly based on the living epitome of Renaissance melancholy, Sir Walter Raleigh, worrying about his risky ventures at sea:

> In sooth I know not why I am so sad,
> It wearies me, you say it wearies you;
> But how I caught it, found it, or came by it,
> What stuff 'tis made of, whereof it is born,
> I am to learn:
> And such a want-wit sadness makes of me,
> That I have much ado to know myself.
>
> (1.1.1–7)

Hamlet confesses that he has 'lost all [his] mirth' and the earth to him seems 'a sterile promontory', a condition which both he and Claudius diagnose as melancholy, Polonius as 'madness'. Each group had its own particular symptoms of melancholy and required individualised treatment according to the unique 'constitution' of each person, sometimes requiring physical intervention like bloodletting or purging. Cures included remedies from a huge range of herbs and minerals chosen on a homeopathic principle of 'like cures like', symptomatised through a larger doctrine of natural 'sympathies', and often rectified by a prescribed change in diet or lifestyle. The study of melancholy was intrinsically holistic. Burton wrote from a belief that body, mind and even soul were integrated, considering that sickness could not be addressed in isolation from the whole, emotional and spiritual being. It is the world of Lady Macbeth's doctor seeking to understand an 'infected mind':

> DOCTOR
>   Not so sick, my Lord,

As she is troubled with thick coming-fancies,
That keep her from her rest.
MACBETH
Cure her of that:
Canst thou not minister to a mind diseas'd,
Pluck from the memory a rooted sorrow,
Raze out the written troubles of the brain,
And with some sweet oblivious antidote
Cleanse the stuff'd bosom of that perilous stuff
Which weighs upon the heart?
DOCTOR
Therein the patient
Must minister to himself.

(5.3.38–45)

This doctor concludes, 'More needs she the divine than the physician', diagnosing her condition as a 'perturbation' of the soul.

Robert Burton

Even writing could help alleviate the condition, at least as a temporary distraction, as Robert Burton self-diagnosed: 'I write of Melancholy, by being busy to avoid Melancholy' (1.6.29–30). There seems little evidence that writing his book succeeded as self-therapy for any length of time, since he kept returning like a dog to a bone to add more authorities and quotations, and an unauthenticated tradition held that he finally committed suicide. His monument in Christ Church Cathedral reads in Latin 'melancholy gave him life and death'. The incongruous saving grace for readers of *The Anatomy of Melancholy* is its unexpectedly rich vein of humour in language, scatological social observations, and idiosyncratic habits of perception, all of which fostered its resurrection among more literary readers after its medical value had fallen away. According to Thomas Warton, eighteenth-century literary scholar, poet laureate, and author of a 'graveyard' poem entitled 'The Pleasures of Melancholy', Milton was also 'an attentive reader of Burton's book', and Warton himself was appreciative of the book's range:

the writer's variety of learning, his quotations from scarce and curious books, his pedantry sparkling with rude wit and shapeless elegance, miscellaneous matter, intermixture of agreeable tales and illustrations, and perhaps above all, the singularities of his feelings cloathed in an uncommon quaintness of style, have contributed to render it, even to modern readers, a valuable repository of amusement and information.[12]

A literary-minded enthusiast writing in 1819 on 'English Writers Compared' in *The Gentleman's Magazine* praises Burton for his 'lively sallies of fancy and imagination' which he says are rare in English prose, quoting a remarkable passage in which Burton describes his digressive style:[13]

> As a long-winged hawk, when he is first whistled off the fist, mounts aloft, and for his pleasure fetcheth many a circuit in the air, still soaring higher and higher, till he be come to his full pitch, and in the end when the game is sprung, comes down amain, and stoops upon a sudden: so will I, having now come at last into these ample fields of air, wherein I may freely expatiate and exercise myself for my recreation, awhile rove, wander round about the world, mount aloft to those ethereal orbs and celestial spheres, and so descend to my former elements again.
>
> (Book 1, Subsec. 2, Memb. 3)

Since this comes in Book 1 of the *Anatomy* we cannot know if Keats read and admired it, but his markings of the next two Books show that he relished to the full these qualities, as we shall see in Chapter 5. He found in Burton's variegated version of melancholy a comprehensive worldview linking his most ever-present preoccupations, Elizabethan literature, poetry, art and medicine, as well as his lived experiences of loss, recurrent grief, and his professional training in the healing art of medicine. We might slightly alter Burton's sentence to describe Keats's stance: 'I *read* of Melancholy, by being busy to avoid Melancholy'. It comes also to be a recurrent theme of his own self-healing poetic writing.

Burton saw melancholy everywhere, not only (in the words of Angus Gowland) as 'the occlusion of reason and the breakdown of psychic harmony in the individual', but also as 'the disintegration of the harmony in society',[14] and to this extent he regarded it as an epidemic with large political, social and religious implications. Intriguingly, some modern scholars in a range of disciplines have speculated that although symptoms change through history, some periods have been especially prone to 'epidemics' of melancholy, citing the Romantic period and even the early twenty-first century, with its apparent growth of anxiety, depression and autism:

> When studying the history of melancholia from ancient times to today, one is dazzled by the chameleonic changes of melancholia, whose definitions vary decisively in different epochs and cultural contexts. Many epochs have been described as particularly prone to melancholia, including our present day – a diagnosis which concerns literature and the arts as well as literary and cultural theory. Andrew Gibson, for instance, sees the 'contemporary aesthetic realm . . . [as] a melancholy space' (136). Julian Schiesari detects a 'rhetoric

of loss' in contemporary cultural theory; and Naomi Schor even diagnoses a general 'melancholy of the disciplines'.[15]

On the other hand, however, even Burton's conclusion about his own period has been challenged, since medical records do not seem to support the epidemic theory in the Renaissance.[16] For example, we see from the casebook of Shakespeare's son-in-law John Hall, who was a practising physician, that he rarely diagnosed melancholy.[17] Such 'epidemical' constructions are probably in the eye of the beholder, and Burton's eye was undoubtedly obsessional, finding melancholy in every nook and cranny of learning, history, society, and individuals. Other more recent scholars of melancholy have accorded it a similarly wide historical ambit, seeing its presence in every generation, as art historian Michael Ann Holly in *The Melancholy Art* documents:

> For many thinkers, the time elapsed between the fourteenth century and the 'end' of modernism in the twentieth represents the era of melancholy, a meta-narrative 'inaugurated by the Renaissance, refined by the Enlightenment, haunted by Romanticism, fetishized by the Decadents, and theorized by Freud' before its reappearance in postmodern critical theory.[18]

Rather than viewing melancholy as periodically being revived in eras separated from each other, it is more persuasive to argue for historical continuity through culturally driven changes and reformulations, from ancient times through to Freud's analysis of melancholia, Kristeva's 'melancholic imaginary', and beyond.

It is clear that in Burton's own era his book was regarded as a work of medical science, and respected as a contribution to what Angus Gowland argues was 'orthodox neo-Galenic university-based medicine' whose methodology, and its textual authorities of 'Hippocratics and Galen, were not displaced from the centre of the curriculum until the 1640s'.[19] In fact, however, the medical education at universities still included the Galenic model and heavily emphasised Latin as the medium of instruction right through to 1815.[20] It seems incredible to us that this approach and such a book as Burton's *Anatomy* could be seen as in any way 'scientific', but until Francis Bacon's empirical method took root, medicine was considered more of an art than a science at the time, and science itself was not viewed as based on observation but reliant on ancient authorities. A glance at the many works on human passions written at the time shows that Burton was synthesising and elaborating on the dominant medical orthodoxy in the Renaissance, which did not sharply separate body, mind, and soul. The publishing history of *The Anatomy of Melancholy* seems to reveal something of its medical reception. Eight editions were printed from 1621 up to 1676, an impressive record for a large and expensive volume. But then there were no more until 1800, with others thereupon following thick and fast, some in one volume and some in two, in 1802, 1806, 1813 (the eleventh edition, which Keats owned), 1821, 1827 and 1838, the last three being reprints of 1813 rather than new editions. *The Anatomy* then fell out of favour again, though from the early twentieth century it has retained a small but dedicated readership in the accessible Everyman reprints. The most obvious explanation for the publishing hiatus from 1676 to 1800, I suggest, would be that up to the mid-seventeenth century it was considered an important compendium of medical knowledge, but once the Galenic model lost currency, and anatomy and surgery came to dominate public hospitals in the eighteenth century, so did scientific respect for Burton's book. Something was lost in this revolution, and it seems to have mattered to Keats, insofar as the older 'patient-centred' art of physicians which paid 'sympathetic' attention to mental states was displaced by more quick-fix results offered by surgery and physical antidotes.[21] It is humbling to reflect that, so steadily does medical research change its methodologies and ideologies, today's 'research' in medicine may similarly be regarded as antiquated and outdated in a hundred years' time.

Although Burton's book lost its medical readership in the eighteenth century (except probably in universities where there were copies in libraries), its revival in 1800 was preceded by important literary figures. Laurence Sterne quoted chunks of Burton in *Tristram Shandy* without acknowledgment. It was admired by Samuel Johnson who, according to Boswell, said 'Burton's *Anatomy of Melancholy* was the only book that ever took him out of bed two hours sooner than he wished to rise'.[22] Having a thought to Johnson's well-documented, lugubrious temperament and fear of insanity, his interest was likely not simply literary, and like Keats later, he had a range of personal motivations driving his interest. He suffered from lifelong bouts of both chronic and acute melancholy, which he explained as a constitution inherited from his father. He felt constantly 'overwhelmed with an horrible melancholia, with perpetual irritation, fretfulness, and impatience; and with a dejection, gloom, and despair, which made existence misery'.[23] He had also in a literary sense inherited from earlier medical authorities a belief that writers especially were predisposed to melancholy. 'Company' was the only temporary cure he found effective, a remedy advocated by most of the earlier authorities, and like Burton he kept himself 'busy' with writing. In his *Dictionary* (1752) he seems still to credit the old Galenic definition, adding two more general meanings, 'A kind of madness, in which the mind is always fixed on one object' and 'A gloomy, pensive, discontented temper'. William Cowper was a literary fellow sufferer in the late eighteenth century, his melancholy so severe that he contemplated suicide.[24] Judging from his constant obsession with having been deserted by God, it seems likely Burton would have diagnosed him as suffering from severe religious melancholy, though a more modern approach would probably point to genetic inheritance as in Johnson's case.

We shall look in more detail below, when we examine Keats's training, at how the radical shift in medical theory came about, but suffice to say at this stage that it comprehensively displaced Burton's approach. As mainstream medicine developed steadily in the eighteenth century towards its modern, allopathic basis (combating disease by administering remedies as antidotes to the condition) and away from the homeopathic model of 'sympathies', so Burton's worldview receded into irrelevance. Surgery became more common as detailed knowledge of the body improved and the professional status of surgeons rose, displacing both the humoural model and the constitutional approach which assumed body and mind were intimately connected. Sir Astley Cooper, Keats's charismatic lecturer at Guy's Hospital, who had himself studied under John Hunter, the eighteenth century pioneer in the study of physiology, anatomy and surgery, was adamant that observation and experimentation, rather than prior authority or non-bodily considerations, ruled supreme in making medical advances:

> In collecting evidence upon any medical subject, there are but three sources from which we can hope to obtain it – from observation on the living subject, from examination of the dead, and from experiments on living animals.[25]

The categorical tone of '*any* medical subject' allowed little room for considering personality, emotions, or mental attributes, thus excluding the possibility of melancholia being a legitimate 'medical' affliction or 'constitutional' state.

There was one small but culturally significant survival, however. By the late eighteenth century the physical effects of disturbance of 'black bile' were medically recognised as 'hypochondrium', located in the abdomen 'under the ribs' (*hypo chondria*) and associated especially with flatuousness in the gall bladder and spleen.[26] Burton had colourfully labelled the illness 'windy melancholy'.[27] The textbooks consulted by Keats in his medical course reveal that hypochondrium was among the subjects he studied.[28] The eighteenth-century medical expert on the physiology of hypochondria was William Cullen at Edinburgh, whose influence extended well into the nineteenth century. However, although hypochondrium in this sense was regarded as a limited and specific physical condition, the word and patients' complaints became increasingly viewed with scepticism by the medical profession. Symptoms were regarded as the product of a delusory mental condition, pointing towards our modern dismissal of 'hypochondriacs', who are regarded as not really having anything wrong with their bodies but are obsessed with imagined illness: 'a morbid state of mind, characterized by general depression, melancholy, or low spirits *for which there is no real cause*' (OED, my italics).[29] Cooper tartly comments in the text book on Anatomy studied by Keats, 'In diseases Medical Men guess, if they cannot ascertain a disease they call it nervous',[30] another word often applied to imaginative writers, as in Keats's 'nervous irritability' above and 'From want of regular rest, I have been rather *narvus*'.[31] With the rise during the eighteenth century of philosophical sentimentalism and its fictional analogue the sentimental novel, both hypochondrium and melancholy fell under the same shadow of disbelief, acquiring cultural and social associations instead of medical. Their reputation grew as an affectation, becoming known as 'the English malady', associated especially with the kind of solitary creativity considered synonymous with Romantic poetry. The phrase had been coined as early as 1733 in the title and subtitle of George Cheyne's *The English Malady: Or, A Treatise of Nervous Diseases of all Kinds*, in which sensibility is signalled as a medical condition of the 'nerves', later in the eyes of unsympathetic reviewers to affect both Della Cruscans, a community of English writers in Florence, and Leigh Hunt's circle which included Keats.[32] The aspersions cast were significantly on political grounds in the 1790s since they were radical.[33] At times some of Keats's own doctors, even his last one, Dr James Clark in Rome, implied his illness was imaginary and the product of a poetic mind. A recent book, *The Age of Hypochondria: Interpreting Romantic Health and Illness* by George C. Grinnell, tells a part of the sorry story in the Romantic age, through case studies of Beddoes, Coleridge, Mary Shelley, de Quincey and other sufferers, though surprisingly he does not mention Keats.[34] Grinnell applies a Foucauldian perspective in attributing the shift to wider, cultural changes, based on seeing illness itself as often an illusion resulting from a regulatory society policing people's quest for physical well-being and perfect body image.

Literary Melancholy: Graveyard Poetry and the Gothic Revival

How, why and in what forms did melancholy (*tristesse* in French literature) become fashionable again among poets in the Romantic period?

One work in particular was hugely influential in regenerating a specific kind of melancholy as a literary subject. The epistolary, semi-autobiographical novel by the German writer, Johann Wolfgang von Goethe *The Sorrows of Young Werther* (1774; translated 1779), swept through Europe like a storm, reputedly causing copy-cat youthful suicides for unrequited love and thwarted creativity. Lord Byron in England capitalised, becoming the first literary 'superstar', when he covered similar emotional terrain in his play *Manfred* (1816–17) depicting a brooding, Faust-like wanderer, and in his long narrative poem *Childe Harold's Pilgrimage* (1812–18). Both established in England Goethe's prototype of the larger-than-life, disillusioned and melancholy wanderer and exemplar of the poet. But this phenomenon sprang from developments in the eighteenth century which, despite its 'enlightenment' faith in reason and a new approach to medicine, persisted in retaining melancholy as a literary category.

Among these was 'graveyard poetry'. Typically the persona, often a poet, would be found at twilight among the tombstones in a graveyard meditating on life and death. Among the first examples was Rev Thomas Parnell's 'A Night Piece on Death' (published 1722):

The left presents a place of graves,
Whose wall the silent water laves.
That steeple guides thy doubtful sight
Among the livid gleams of night.
There pass, with melancholy state,
By all the solemn heaps of fate,
And think, as softly-sad you tread
Above the venerable dead.[35]

Elizabeth Carter's 'Ode to Melancholy', 'A Night-Piece' and 'Thoughts at Midnight' (1730s) all owed something to Milton's quietly meditative 'Il Penseroso'. Next in influence, and different in atmosphere, came the lengthier poem 'The Grave' (1743) by the Scottish Robert Blair (who, like Parnell, also became a minister),[36] which was illustrated by Blake in 1808. The self-appointed task of the poet, he proposes, is 'To paint the gloomy horrors of the tomb ... The Grave, dread thing!'. The more sensational imagery, with its 'horrid apparition' and the screams of 'night's foul bird | Rook'd in the spire' derived from *Macbeth* and *Hamlet*, points towards the coming Gothic revival. Edward Young's 'Night Thoughts' (in full, 'The Complaint: or, Night-Thoughts on Life, Death, & Immortality)' (1742–5), also illustrated by Blake (1797), was more ambitious, tracing over nine painful nights the emotional meditations of the grief-stricken poet who has lost his wife:

> How populous, how vital, is the grave!
> This is creation's melancholy vault,
> The vale funereal, the sad cypress gloom;
> The land of apparitions, empty shades![37]

The most famous example is the more calmly introspective 'Elegy Written in a Country Churchyard' (1751) by Thomas Gray, an influential model for Romantic literary conventions of melancholy, and yet again engraved by Blake. In a state of 'lonely contemplation' the poet muses on the varied lives which had been led by all those who lie dead in the graveyard, from lowly nonentities to petty tyrants. These include an archetypally lovelorn young poet, described on his epitaph as one whom 'Melancholy marked . . . for her own': 'He gave to Misery all he had, a tear'.[38] We are reminded that, in Shakespeare's words in one of the first examples of graveyard poetry, 'Golden lads and lasses must, like chimney-sweepers come to dust'.[39] The poet writing the elegy transparently envisages his own ultimate fate, and generalises on the vanity of wishes when death comes to all. Almost as famous as Gray's 'Elegy' and reprinted into the Romantic age, was Thomas Warton the Younger's lengthy *The Pleasures of Melancholy*, published as a pamphlet in 1747. Its celebrity perhaps owed most to the author's precocity since he was only seventeen when he first wrote it, but the soporifically meditative poem has not fared so well as Gray's:

> O lead me, black-brow'd Queen, to solemn glooms
> Congenial with my soul, to chearless shades,
> To ruin'd seats, to twilight cells and bow'rs,
> Where thoughtful Melancholy loves to muse,
> Her fav'rite midnight haunts.[40]

'The Pleasures of Melancholy' was based clearly on Milton's 'Il Penseroso' which in its mood at least could be claimed as the genre's prototype, and as mentioned, Warton admired Burton's book and detected its influence behind Milton's poetry as a whole. Surveying the spectrum from Blair and Young through to the soulful musings of Warton, Carter and Gray reveals the breadth of melancholy in the process of being transferred from medicine into graveyard poetry, changing from an affliction of body, soul and mind into an inward, mental construct, a free-floating emotion stimulated in a suggestively mournful environment focused on death.

Owing something in outlook to graveyard poetry, Coleridge's 'Dejection: An Ode' (written 1802) describes a more psychologically based and emotional state of 'dull pain': 'A grief without a pang, void, dark, and drear, I A stifled, drowsy, unimpassioned grief'. The poet can 'see, not feel' the beauty around him, and in this state of alienation he cannot 'hope from outward forms to win | The passion and the life, whose fountains are within'. The 'Ode' then follows a therapeutic path on 'wings of healing', as the poet strives to recapture lost 'Joy' through his 'shaping spirit of Imagination' in order to recover the capacity to write.[41] The loosening of his 'viper thoughts' comes spontaneously, as a combination of love and identification with living things and natural processes, bringing about a peaceful closure to a poem which, in a suggestive phrase used by William Hazlitt, charts a 'logic of passion' conducted through writing of melancholy.

Graveyard poetry contributed to another increasingly fashionable, affectively defined genre, the Gothic novel, initiated in *The Castle of Otranto* (1764) by Horace Walpole, presented as a medieval revival and popularising a 'cult of ruins'. Wealthy landowners in England were drawn to erecting ruins in their grounds, sometimes even housing in them a poet as a kind of melancholy writer-in-residence. The genre built upon fictionalised externalisations of the inner landscape of melancholy: a mysterious castle, pervading atmosphere of ominous foreboding and palpable evil, and an emphasis on heightened emotional states of fear and horror.[42] Keats fused melancholy and Gothic conventions in *The Eve of St. Agnes, Isabella*, and 'Ode on Melancholy', and he parodies himself in a letter before his Scottish journey with Brown:

> I am going among Scenery whence I intend to rip you the Damosel Radcliffe – I'll cavern you, and grotto you, and waterfall you, and wood you, and water you, and immense-rock you, and tremendous sound you, and solitude you. Ill make a lodgement on glacis by a row of Pines, and storm your covered way with Bramble bushes . . .[43]

Keats also jokes about the 'fine mother Radcliff names' of his own works: 'the Pot of Basil, St Agnes eve, and if I should have finished it a little thing call'd "the eve of St Mark"'.[44] The Gothic genre was regarded as especially aimed at female readers, and some women wrote examples, including Ann Radcliffe's *The Mysteries of Udolpho* (1794), Charlotte Smith's novels and poetry, and Mary Shelley's *Frankenstein; or, The Modern Prometheus* (1818). It was also a woman, Jane Austen (1775–1817), who sought to puncture the Gothic novel's hypnotic hold over credulous readers, personified in Catherine Morland in *Northanger Abbey* (1818), which gently debunks the conventions of a fictional genre regarded as being consumed avidly by a young, 'immature and uninformed' audience.[45] In similar vein, Thomas Love Peacock (1785–1866) in his hilarious novels *Headlong Hall* (1815) and *Nightmare Abbey* (1818) satirised his poetic friends, Coleridge, Shelley and Byron, for their self-conscious dedication to melancholia. However, by the 1820s, as Jane Austen's *Northanger Abbey* foreshadowed, the Gothic version of melancholy was becoming a fashionable pose among the wealthy and literati. Keats, like Austen and Peacock, could satirise the sentimental movement's passing vogue in his 'nonsense verses' written on 17 September, 1819, 'Pensive they sit, and roll their languid eyes'. He ridicules 'Mr Werter' using his inverted spoon to rescue a drowning fly from the milk pot: 'must he die | Circled by a Humane Society?'. Although his main targets are the oversensitive members of the Royal Humane Society, yet the name of 'Mr. Werter' recalls Goethe's titular hero. A lifelong sufferer from his own acute sympathetic melancholy, he could yet see through the fakeries of the new-fashioned *poseur*.

It was in this climate of melancholy sensibility that Burton's *Anatomy of Melancholy* was rediscovered, this time as a literary phenomenon. Coleridge annotated the book, Wordsworth, Green, and Southey owned copies, as did Keats's artist friend Haydon. Byron praised it on literary grounds, and Charles Lamb was an outright enthusiast. In America Herman Melville in 1847 bought an 1821 'selected' edition.[46] We can thank both Coleridge and Charles Lamb for reviving interest in Burton's book, after a blank period from publication of the eighth edition in 1676 to 1800, during which there was no new edition.[47] Lamb owned a first edition, published in 1621, and wrote jovially to Thomas Manning on 17 March, 1800, about his plan to produce 'the forgery of a supposed manuscript of Burton that anatomist of melancholy':

> [Coleridge] has lugged me to the brink of engaging to a newspaper, and has suggested to me for a first plan the forgery of a supposed manuscript of Burton the anatomist of melancholy. I have even written the introductory letter; and, if I can pick up a few guineas this way, I feel they will be most *refreshing*, bread being so dear.[48]

The odd project of 'forging' or imitating Burton reached neither the publisher which Lamb courted, nor a conclusion, but examples appeared among 'Curious Fragments' in Lamb's *John Woodvill: A Tragedy* (1802). Lamb described them as 'extracted from a commonplace book, which belonged to Robert Burton, the famous Author of The Anatomy of Melancholy'.[49] He expanded on the nature of Burton's writing in another letter to Manning on 5 April:

> I had struck off two imitations of Burton, quite abstracted from any modern allusions, which it was my intent only to lug in from time to time to make 'em popular. ... Burton is a scarce gentleman, not much known; else I had done 'em pretty well.
> I have also hit off a few lines in the name of Burton, being a conceit of

'Diabolic Possession.' Burton was a man often assoiled by deepest melancholy, and at other times much given to laughing and jesting, as is the way with melancholy men. I will send them you: they were almost extempore, and no great things; but you will indulge them.[50]

However, the more important result of Lamb's intense interest in the work was the republication in 1800 of Robert Burton's *The Anatomy of Melancholy* itself in its ninth edition. Even if Lamb did not fulfil his own quixotic project, he helped spark a revival and inspired new readers, among whom was Keats.

In other words, by the Romantic age the reception and readership of Burton had changed from predominantly medical to entirely literary. Keats was the only one to have a professional foot in both fields and could read it as both a poet, and as a doctor professionally aware of its historical medical context. By his time, medicine had not fully abandoned all its idealism and ancient knowledge which was consolidated in the vast and ever-growing *materia medica,* listing remedies for symptoms, which constituted a significant part of the syllabus at Guy's Hospital. For Keats, the older medical context and surviving vocabulary would have been at least familiar to him, especially with his school days' expertise in Latin (also essential for medical training), while Burton's writing held the same literary allure for him as for some of his contemporaries. In addition, more so than any of his poetic contemporaries, Keats's literary affinities lay firmly in the Renaissance: the world of Spenser, Shakespeare, Milton, and Burton.

Keats: Poetry, Melancholy, and Healing

From early on Keats was well aware of his own congenital tendency to melancholy, describing it to Haydon in this way:

You tell me never to despair – I wish it was as easy for me to observe the saying – truth is I have a horrid Morbidity of Temperament which has shown itself at intervals – it is I have no doubt the greatest Enemy and stumbling block I have to fear – I may even say that it is likely to be the cause of my disappointment.[51]

He had ample cause for such moods in his own life experiences, and he could regard the state as by turns an affliction, a source of medical study, and a creative stimulus. It became a frequent facet of his poetry expressing a temperamental 'hateful siege of contraries'[52] – a phrase directly quoted from Milton's *Paradise Lost* (9.121):

I must choose between despair & Energy – I choose the latter – though the
world has taken on a quakerish look with me, which I once thought was
impossible –
    'Nothing can bring back the hour
    Of splendour in the grass and glory in the flower'
I once thought this a Melancholist's dream – [53]

He often thought about the potential for generating his own unique
body of creative work from his fluctuating emotions, envisaging 'a kind
of Pleasure Thermometer' which would help in his 'chief Attempt in the
Drama – the playing of different Natures with Joy and Sorrow'.[54] The
phrase 'the playing of different Natures with Joy and Sorrow' could
stand as an apt description of the 1820 collection.

There were many points in Keats's life when wounds of loss were
inflicted. Even allowing for abbreviated life expectancy at the time
(under 40), he had ample reason for suffering almost constant grief in
his early years as he faced mortality in his family. He was to write to
Fanny Brawne, 'I have never known any unalloy'd Happiness for many
days together: the death or sickness of some one has always spoilt my
hours'.[55] Among the 'significant others' he lost were a one-year-old
brother, Edward, when John was five; his father, Thomas, at eight; and
his mother, Frances, when John was fifteen, thus orphaning him and his
siblings. The losses of his parents both occurred when he was at board-
ing school, and provoked erratic behaviour in the schoolboy. During the
absence of his mother, his grandmother Alice Jennings became virtually
a surrogate mother to the Keats children, and she then died when he was
nineteen. At twenty-three his brother Tom died, after being supported
and nursed for months by John. An uncle Midgley also died in Keats's
lifetime, and perhaps other relatives and school friends. Added to such
devastating losses by death were other kinds of traumatic separation,
such as apparent abandonment by his widowed mother and her sudden
marriage to William Rawlings just two months later. In adulthood, Keats
sometimes compared himself to Hamlet, and it must have haunted him
to reflect that he shared the same fate of losing his father and acquiring a
stepfather in the same short time frame. He was also disconcerted by the
apparently precipitate emigration of his newly married brother George
to America, and by periods of absence from both his beloved younger
sister Fanny when she was the ward of Abbey, and enforced isolation
through his illness from his fiancée Fanny Brawne at important stages of
their relationship. Omnipresent also in his consciousness as time went
on were anxieties about money, and the gathering premonitions of his
own premature death from tuberculosis, just as he was rapidly develop-
ing his poetic powers: an immeasurably intense sense of imminent loss,

anticipated even in early poems. A different, though equally shattering, 'disappointment' came with the devastating critical reception of his first two books. Especially cruel was the onslaught on *Endymion* by Lockhart writing under the name of 'Z' in *Blackwood's Edinburgh Quarterly*. He noted with personal venom the poet's 'career of medicine ... bound apprentice some years ago to a worthy apothecary in town'. The reviewer sarcastically advised him, 'It is a better and a wiser thing to be a starved apothecary than a starved poet; so back to the shop Mr. John, "back to the plaster, pills and ointment boxes," &c ... be a little more sparing of extenuatives and soporifics in your practice than you have been in your poetry'.[56] Save for Keats's resilient self-belief in his poetry, this could have constituted the loss of his aspirations before they had been realised, and such attacks became mythologised after his death as the cause of his demise.

Freud, in his analysis of the difference between acute grief which eventually passes ('mourning') and chronic 'melancholia' emphasises in particular the significance of the loss of the mother, whether by death, indifference or abandonment, as an infantile experience which can unconsciously be reactivated by loss in later life.[57] Jennifer Radden suggests, 'Adult melancholia at the least mimics, but perhaps even re-enacts, the psychic incorporation of the mother by the infant' which at some stage is lost.[58] In what may be a glancing memory of his mother, Keats ascribes his discomfort in the company of women to 'being disappointed since Boyhood'.[59] Freud's analysis seems to suggest that Keats's frequent and periodic mourning, especially over his mother's disappearance from the family and then her death, deepened into a more serious and chronic state of melancholia.

There is plenty of evidence in his letters and poems that Keats suffered bouts of extreme self-criticism, self-devaluation and 'self-reproaches', all conditions described by Freud (p. 248) as responses to loss as 'the wound [laceration] that never heals', stretching well past his understandable self-consciousness due to his diminutive height. Most unusual are sensations of losing his identity when in company, feelings of personal dissolution and self-annihilation implicit in his theory of 'Negative Capability', and his reports of lapsing into 'horrid morbidity'. The bipolar fluctuation between despair and mania exhibited in his sonnet, 'Why did I laugh tonight? No voice will tell' recounts a kind of oscillating melancholy which had been described by Timothy Bright as 'unbridled laughter' not aroused by 'gladness of spirit' but instead as a kind of 'counterfeit' masking the melancholy.[60] Keats's cry from 'the human heart' of being 'here sad and alone', is ruptured by sudden and inexplicable laughter in the midst of a chasm of 'Darkness! Darkness!', followed by an embrace of the intensity of death – 'Death is Life's high meed'. The state of mind revealed in this sonnet alarmed Keats himself, to the extent that he felt driven to reassure the recipients of his letter, his brother George and sister-in-law Georgiana, not to worry about him: 'I am ever afraid that your anxiety for me will lead you to fear for the violence of my temperament continually smothered down: for that reason I did not intend to have sent you the following sonnet ...'. But asserting his mental resilience, he concludes, 'Sane I went to bed and sane I arose' (March 1819). In May 1818 he had complained to Bailey of a 'Lethargy', and of feeling 'so depressed that I have not an Idea to put to paper – my hand feels like lead – and yet it is an[d] unpleasant numbness it does not take away the pain of existence'. He adds that his 'intellect must be in a degen[er]ating state', worried about troubling Bailey with 'Moods of my own Mind or rather body – for mind there is none. I am in that temper that if I were under Water I would scarcely kick to come to the top.'[61] 'Ode to a Nightingale' traces a similar mental dissolution in the desire to 'Fade far away, dissolve, and quite forget ...', followed by 'I have been half in love with easeful Death' when 'Now more than ever seems it rich to die'. The sequence of feelings depicted in the ode provides an extraordinary description of psychological symptoms as the poem simultaneously describes and even relishes the falling into and out of oblivion. Through the medium of poetry, Keats recreates, contemplates and chronicles his sense of almost continual loss causing mourning and deeper melancholia, as he seeks to transcend the feelings through the self-healing medium of poetry.

Keats's Medical Training[62]

Keats's training as surgeon-apothecary sharpened his awareness and understanding of physical and mental suffering, and was also formative in his view of the functions of poetry as a healing agent in alleviating pain. It is possible that there was a line of medical professionals on Keats's father's side of the family, but evidently his actual decision to study medicine came either during, or as a consequence of, his attentiveness to caring for his mother during her fatal illness, and as a response to her death. Almost immediately in 1810 he became apprenticed to the local Edmonton medical practitioner, Thomas Hammond, who was qualified as both apothecary and surgeon, as Keats was to be. As the next step, in October 1815 he entered Guy's Hospital, officially known as the United Hospitals of Guy's and St Thomas's in London. He was rapidly 'promoted' to the responsible role of dressership at Guy's, suggesting that he was among the best students in the cohort. However, by the time he graduated in July 1816 as a fully qualified surgeon-apothecary, he had resolved to earn his living as a poet. In the eyes of his guardian Richard Abbey, who controlled the purse-strings of the Keats siblings' inheritance which had paid for his training, medicine seemed like an expensive false start, but in fact the training was to clarify and reinforce his attitude to poetry as a healing medium. As he put it when he was writing 'Isabella', his 'Bias' in infancy became 'no Bias': 'Every department of knowledge we see excellent and calculated towards a great whole. I am so convinced of this, that I am glad at not having given away my medical Books'.[63] It chimed with a temperamentally altruistic desire to use 'Knowledge' to pursue 'the idea of doing some good for the world',[64] and also supported his own, apparently self-diagnosing and ongoing identification with melancholy. The 'Knowledge' he gained in his training as a medical student was undoubtedly sobering and often horrifying. In the working environment at Guy's Hospital, he was made acutely aware of the pathological significance of melancholy and madness in all their varied forms. Not only was there the extreme physical suffering of poverty-stricken patients in excruciating pain, but there were also wards filled with patients with dementia, historically considered as extreme melancholia, and young people dying of consumption.

Keats had entered Guy's Hospital in a year of profound change to the medical profession, arriving at the same time as the final, though qualified, success of a long campaign to legislate the Apothecaries Act in 1815.[65] The Act marked a series of radical changes in medical practice over the late eighteenth century, as the result of a power struggle between the two dominant branches of the profession: surgeons and physicians. The tensions were brought to a head by the disastrous shortcomings starkly exposed in the almost nonexistent national medical services on the bloody fields after the Battle of Waterloo in 1815. The far-reaching significance of the Act can be seen in terms of its effects on Keats's own experience. As a result of the institutional victory of surgeons and the rise of public hospitals, the basis for a hegemony of the Royal College of Surgeons was emerging at just the time Keats entered Guy's. Roy Porter sums up by saying that there was 'a shift from a physiological theory (disease is an abnormal condition of the whole organism) to an ontological theory of disease (disease is an entity residing locally in a part) . . . Pathology had now been put, alongside anatomy, on a scientific footing'.[66] Some would add darkly to these words, 'for better or worse' and among them, I believe, would be Keats. It does seem likely that he was attracted to the older, humanistic and integrated model of medicine exemplified by Burton, and averse to the new developments in anatomy and surgery, which separated the part from the whole, and the body from the mind or soul.[67] By this stage he had resolved to make poetry his profession, and it is surprising to see how many poems he had already written while a medical student.[68]

In earlier times, being an apothecary was to belong to what was described in a book published in 1747 by R. Campbell, *The London Tradesman*, as 'a Profession that requires very little Brains', merely a 'strong Memory, to retain such a Number of Cramp Words as he is daily conversant with'.[69] This was despite the fact that, to all but the rich who could afford a physician, the apothecary was no doubt of far more use to the general health of the community than the lofty physician. By means of the 1815 Act, however, the importance of the apothecary in public medicine was recognised as the first step on the professional ladder that could lead higher. This was because the 'winners' of the professional dispute, the surgeons, tied apothecary apprentices to their own claims for advancement in status, allowing for the apothecary first to ascend to the ranks of surgeons through internship at a teaching hospital. The victory was over the group traditionally heading the hierarchy, namely conservative Oxbridge graduates who belonged to the ancient Royal College of Physicians (founded in 1518) and had always monopolised the coveted title of 'physician'. Their training was still close to the clois-tered university world of Burton's medical authority.[70] Apothecaries, like surgeons, benefited from the Act, since their previously disrespected status and minimal training were substantially upgraded. Keats per-sonally benefited in a professional sense. Having begun pre-1815 as a humble apprentice apothecary in Enfield, debarred from university entrance since he was from a dissenting family, he found his final quali-fication to be effectively that of a novice surgeon, analogous to our general practitioner, with the possibility of rising even higher. The term 'general practitioner' itself was being used by Keats's time for the quali-fied apothecary.[71]

In Campbell's account, the surgeon in the early eighteenth century had dealt only with externalities like wounds, bruises, ulcers, venereal diseases and 'Eruptions in the outward Parts', requiring mainly manual dexterity and an ability 'not to give way to Pity and Compassion' in per-forming amputations. Surgery had historically been practised by barbers (perhaps because they had the sharpest knives?) but these trades had been separated just a year before Campbell wrote. In their newfound professional independence, surgeons at this stage were mainly destined for serving in the navy as ships' doctors. By 1800 their Royal College was established, rivalling that of the Physicians.[72] Their status had improved with the growing paradigm shift to anatomy and surgery and the rise of the public hospital system. A part of what Keats retained from his time at Guy's was embodied in the paradoxical attitude of the famous surgeon-lecturer, Sir Astley Cooper, who personally knew, supported and encouraged Keats, 'going out of his way to assist Keats in finding accommodation and probably also helping to secure his dressership',[73] a role carrying considerable responsibility. Surgeons were trained to focus exclusively on physical symptomology and treatment, since this was considered more commensurate with the (literally) cutting edge scientific method of the day. Cooper, who epitomised this approach, had little time for feelings in his own practice, as his biographer notes:

> If a patient was too frightened to submit, he felt, it was the surgeon's respon-sibility to get the job done. He was brutal, insensitive to physical pain and a bully. He was also devotedly compassionate. He had watched surgeons (including his uncle) shy away from essential operations, too frightened by the horror of performing them. Such actions, he argued, were unjustifiable. The world was full of pain, and anyone who wanted to make it a better place – particularly with a scalpel – had best have the stomach for it. He seemed to find this easy. Physical suffering made little immediate impression on him, and he was so far from being revolted by operating as to actively enjoy it.[74]

'Devotedly compassionate' and driven to make the world a better place, but lacking in squeamishness and probably empathy, Cooper epitomised the paradoxes and contradictions Keats was driven to explore. But by the time he graduated, he seemed out of sympathy with the contemporary fashion for surgery and anatomy, evidenced in the students' guide that he was given on entering Guy's,[75] and in the stern practice of Cooper. Charles Brown reported later,

> He ascribes his inability [to operate] to an overwrought apprehension of every possible chance of doing evil in the wrong direction of the instrument. 'My last operation', he told me, 'was the opening of a man's temporal artery. I did it with the utmost nicety; but reflecting on what passed through my mind at the time, my dexterity seemed a miracle, and I never took up the lancet again.[76]

Nicholas Roe suggests he may have been the duty surgeon under the name of 'Mr Keats' who removed a pistol-ball from the head of one Jane Hull on 25 March 1816.[77] Despite his 'dexterity', Keats's response to the harrowing conditions of dissections of the rotting dead and amputations of the living in the operating theatre in days before anaesthesia was never to take up the lancet again, and instead turn to poetry as his voca-tion. I have argued elsewhere that his decision not to pursue medicine as a career was based partly on a realisation that he was increasingly out of sympathy with the contemporary concentration on anatomy and surgery in experimental teaching hospitals.[78] Given his close encounter with his own immediate teacher at Guy's, the incompetent, swashbuckling surgeon Billy Lucas, it would not be at all surprising if he hankered for older notions of constitutional and herbal healing reminiscent of Burton's day, tending to the mind as much as the body, in the 'bedside encounters' described by Roy Porter:

> We need to question medical history's preoccupying concern with cures (even cures that don't work). It is modern medicine that is cure-fixated. Pharmaceutical intervention in the past ... paid great attention to pain control, to fortifying the body, to adjusting the whole constitution. And treatment went far beyond drug interventions, involving complex rituals of comfort and condolence, the consolations of philosophy and grit, acted out by the suffering, with the physician sometimes sharing in the psycho-dynamics of the bedside encounter.[79]

He continued to ponder how the genuine poet as distinct from the poetic 'dreamer' might, equally unflinchingly, face up to the task of healing psychic and emotional pain, not with the scalpel, but with a constitutional attentiveness to the whole person, including the sickness of the mind as well as the body: '"sure a poet is a sage, | "A humanist, physician to all men"' (*The Fall of Hyperion. A Dream*).

This conception of the poet-healer was closer to the position at the apex of the traditional medical professions, the 'Physician', described by Campbell as a university graduate who had learned his profession from books, especially Galen, rather than experimentation – in other words in its old-fashioned Oxbridge ethos a world away from the ambience of Guy's Hospital. It represented not only the intellectual environment of Burton but also quite likely the image of a doctor to which the young Keats aspired when he chose the profession. Campbell was as stern as Cooper but with a completely different emphasis. His discrimination between good and bad physicians did not lie in the ability to inflict pain without flinching, but in gifts of humane cultivation:

> The Physician, if learned and conscientious, has the Honour to practise a Profession the most useful to Society, and in *England* the most profitable to himself, of any that is affected by human Learning; whereas, if he is ignorant, conceited, or self-interested, he no sooner commences Doctor than he becomes a Plague to Society, an Enemy of Mankind, and a Scandal to his Profession. (p. 37)

He amplifies,

> But let the Physician be both learned and experienced, yet he is still useless, nay hurtful, to Society, unless he has a large Share of Honesty and Humanity ... whose Soul is fired with Charity, Love, and universal Benevolence towards

Mankind . . . such a man is an Ornament to his Profession, and an useful Member of Society . . . In my opinion, the Doctor must be born, not made, as well as the Poet, or Painter: He must have a natural Turn of Mind to the Healing Art . . .

(42–3)

The bar is set high – 'His Education must be Liberal, improv'd both by the study of Men and Books, which he must finish by Travel into Foreign Countries' (p. 44) – after which he can be admitted into the Royal College of Physicians and become 'a legitimate Son of *Aesculapius*' (p. 46). This equated with earning high salaries, tending to the wealthy in their homes. After qualifying as surgeon-apothecary Keats did consider going further:

I have been at different times turning in my head whether I should go to Edinburgh & study for a physician; I am afraid I should not take kindly to it, I am sure I could not take fees – & yet I should like to do so . . .[80]

It had to be Edinburgh, since his nonconformist family background debarred him from English universities (which is why he went to Guy's), and Scotland did not owe allegiance to the Church of England. Timothy Ziegenhagen, in his very thorough article, 'Keats, Professional Medicine, and the Two Hyperions', argues that Keats's true aspiration in the medical profession was to become a physician, attributing this mainly to a desire for the status of a 'gentleman'.[81] But given his reluctance to 'take fees', I suggest his main aim was to acquire the 'knowledge enormous' that could distinguish him as the kind of compassionate 'humanist, physician to all men', alongside the part of the medical profession that was historically aligned with literary knowledge and could genuinely 'heal' hurt minds, one who 'pours out a balm' upon humanity. He was well aware of the classical Apollo's role as patron of medicine and poetry alike, linking poetry and healing; his own chosen, apparently lifelong, mission, from the early 'Sleep and Poetry' to the late *The Fall of Hyperion. A Dream*. Other Romantics also explored the terrain of poetry and healing, as Brittany Pladek demonstrates in her recent book, *The Poetics of Palliation: Romantic Literary Therapy, 1790–1850*,[82] but none was so uniquely qualified as Keats. He was never to relinquish fully what he had learned of melancholy and suffering in his medical vocation, and he turned his knowledge and aspirations to poetic ends.

The true legacy of Keats's medical training was to lie not in the world of doctors, but of psychiatrists. So far as I know there is no evidence that Freud ever read Keats, though he was constantly making reference to Shakespeare, whose works the poet had also deeply absorbed, and upon which in many ways he had modelled his own ideas of the 'poetic identity'. However, one psychiatrist whose works have become almost as influential as Freud's was the British practitioner, Wilfred Bion, and his particular awakening came through encountering Keats's idea of 'Negative Capability':

> that is, when a man is capable of being in uncertainties, mysteries, doubts, without any irritable reaching after fact and reason – Coleridge, for instance, would let go by a fine isolated verisimilitude caught from the Penetralium of mystery, from being incapable of remaining content with half-knowledge.[83]

Bion was deeply struck, as in an epiphany, by Keats's description when treating shell-shocked soldiers in a military hospital during the Second World War, and thereafter it deeply influenced his own clinical practice and theoretical explorations. He cultivated and advocated a nonjudgmental openness to experience, including suffering, tolerating a high degree of ambiguity by living and listening in the present moment, striving 'to impose on himself a positive discipline of eschewing memory and desire' and premature judgment.[84] However, one critic suggests that in Bion's understanding 'Negative Capability' is subtly different from Keats's usage, prioritising 'retroactive' deferment of interpretation rather than 'a learned comfort with the limits of one's curiosity': that is to say, Bion advocates postponing judgment rather than eliminating it altogether.[85] Nonetheless, he explicitly acknowledges that his primary source is Keats's passage, which is itself wonderfully open to interpretation and application in a variety of contexts. Bion was also to work with Melanie Klein, whose approach to working with children traumatised by loss through 'projective identification' was to help him develop his concepts. Others more recently have followed Bion's lead, incorporating Keats into therapeutic practice, among them psychotherapist Diana Voller in several articles which see Keats's concept as offering a 'mode of inhabiting uncertainty', with 'X-factor' defined as 'a term for the unknown factor . . . in which the only certainty is uncertainty'.[86] Bion's approach has become influential, not only in modern psychoanalysis and psychotherapy,[87] but also social work[88] and even business management theory.[89] To Keats goes the credit.

Furthermore, the unique stance of Keats, as simultaneously a suffering patient and aspiring to be a healing physician, has also been found to be useful in personal ways in coping with modern manifestations of mental illness, as equivalents of the earlier melancholy. In a recent book by a Romantic specialist, *How to Make a Soul: The Wisdom of John Keats*, Eric G. Wilson movingly recounts his own experiences of overcoming chronic depression by living empathetically through the life and writings of Keats, finding there an 'addiction to learning' which can turn the negative into positive:

> This is the conversion of depression into melancholy: sullenness over what's gone into yearning for what can come, apathy into somber hope, the limbo of mere lethargy, 'no one thing is better than anything else,' to the limbo of readiness: 'everything, potentially, is interesting'.
>
> That is what melancholy for Keats (and now for me), is: not, again, depression, but a hunger for more life, so intense that the object longed for becomes more vivid than if possessed.[90]

There is, then, more at stake than mere literary antiquarianism in analysing the Keatsian self-healing capacity to turn the negative into positive, in the poems in *1820*, culminating especially in 'Ode on Melancholy'. Melancholy confronted Keats at every turn, through emotional predisposition, devastating family losses, concentrated medical training, as a literary trope evolving through the Renaissance and eighteenth century into Romanticism, and as a cultural concept which had changed from ancient times to his own day. Reading Burton's *Anatomy of Melancholy* in 1819 drew together many of these preoccupations of medicine, melancholy, poetry, and literature. Ian Jack makes a high claim which I hope to substantiate: 'All the . . . Odes of Keats could well be annotated from *The Anatomy of Melancholy* (which was one of Keats's favourite books)' (p. 234). To Keats's animated reading of this book we now turn.

Notes

1. Nicholas Roe, *John Keats*, pp. 16, 273–4.
2. *Oxford English Dictionary* online (hereafter *OED*), 'psychology' 2b.
3. See Sullivan, *Beyond Melancholy: Sadness and Selfhood in Renaissance England*.
4. Gowland, 'Melancholy, Imagination, and Dreaming in Renaissance Learning', pp. 54–102, 56.
5. Jackson, p. 31.
6. To Fanny Keats, 21 April 1820, *LJK*, 2, p. 287.
7. Fitzpatrick, p. 3.
8. Klibansky, Panofsky and Saxl, *Saturn and Melancholy: Studies in the History of Natural Philosophy, Religion and Art*.
9. Dixon, pp. 435–50.
10. See Andrea Bubenik (ed.), *Five Centuries of Melancholia*.
11. For a full coverage, see Bernard, *Shakespearean Melancholy: Philosophy, Form, and the Transformation of Comedy*.
12. John Milton, *Poems Upon Several Occasions*, ed. Thomas Warton, p. 94.
13. *The Gentleman's Magazine* 89 (1819), p. 599.

14. Gowland, *The Worlds of Renaissance Melancholy: Robert Burton in Context*, p. 17.
15. Middeke and Wald (eds), p. 1. Citations from Gibson, pp. 123–41; Julian Schiesari, *The Gendering of Melancholia: Feminism, Psychoanalysis, and the Symbolics of Loss in Renaissance Literature*; and Schor, *One Hundred Years of Melancholy*. See also Enderwitz, *Modernist Melancholia: Freud, Conrad and Ford*.
16. Gowland, 'The Problem of Early Modern Melancholy', pp. 77–120.
17. John Hall, *John Hall and his Patients*.
18. Michael Ann Holly, p. 8.
19. Gowland, *The Worlds of Renaissance Melancholy*, p. 54.
20. Rivlin, pp. 56–63, 56–7.
21. Porter, 'The Patient's View: Doing Medical History from Below', pp. 175–98.
22. Boswell, i, p. 389.
23. Bate, *Samuel Johnson*, p. 117; quoted Jackson, p. 142.
24. Jackson, pp. 137–9.
25. Quoted in Cooper, 'The Hunterian Oration on Astley Cooper and Hunterian Principles', p. 361.
26. See Haskell, 'The Anatomy of Hypochondria' in *Diseases of the Imagination*, pp. 275–300, 56–7.
27. Burton, First Part, Sec. 3, Memb. 2, Subsect. 2.
28. Jackson, pp. 124–9.
29. Goellnicht, pp. 173–4 quotes contemporary medical sources.
30. Keats, *John Keats's Anatomical and Physiological Note Book*, ed. Maurice Buxton Forman, p. 57.
31. To Reynolds, 17–18 April 1817, *LJK*, p. 132.
32. See Clucas, pp. 122–36.
33. See Chris Jones, *Radical Sensibility: Literature and Ideas in the 1790s*; Jon Mee, pp. 104–22; and R. S. White, *Natural Rights and the Birth of Romanticism in the 1790s*, pp. 63–76.
34. Grinnell, *The Age of Hypochondria: Interpreting Romantic Health and Illness*.
35. Parnell, p. 93.
36. Parisot, *Graveyard Poetry* examines the importance of melancholy in the genre. See also Mark, *Marked by melancholy*.
37. Young, p. 5.
38. Greenblatt, *Norton Anthology*, p. 305.
39. *Cymbeline*, 4.2.
40. Warton, *The Pleasures of Melancholy: A Poem*, pp. 4–5.
41. Greenblatt, *Norton Anthology*, p. 479.
42. Hughes, Punter and Smith, 1, pp. 304–5.
43. To Reynolds, 14 March 1818, *LJK*, p. 245.
44. To George Keatses, 14 Feb. onwards 1819, *LJK*, p. 62.
45. Reyes, p. 20.
46. For the title page signed by Melville <http://melvillesmarginalia.org/Popup.aspx?fn=2> (last accessed 20 March 2020)
47. For full history and descriptions of the different editions up to 1651, see Dodsworth, 1, pp. xxxvii–lxi.

48. Charles and Mary Lamb, *Letters*, V, pp. 159–60.
49. Charles and Mary Lamb, *Miscellaneous Prose*, I, p. 35.
50. Charles and Mary Lamb, *Miscellaneous Prose*, V, p. 161.
51. To Haydon, 10, 11 May 1817, *LJK*, 1, p. 141.
52. To Dilke 20 September 1818, *LJK*, 1, pp. 368–9.
53. To Mary-Ann Jeffery, 31 March 1819, quoting Wordsworth, 'Ode: Intimations of Immortality', ll. 180–1.
54. To Taylor, 30 January 1818, *LJK* 2, p. 219.
55. To Fanny Brawne, 1 July, 1819, *LJK*, 2, p. 123.
56. 'Z', 'The Cockney School of Poetry, no. iv', *Blackwood's Edinburgh Magazine*, 3 (1818) 519–24, 519.
57. Freud, *The Standard Edition of the Complete Psychological Works of Sigmund Freud*, xiv (1914–18).
58. Radden, *Moody Minds Distempered: Essays on Melancholy and Depression*, pp. 147–65. See also Radden's *The Nature of Melancholy from Aristotle to Kristeva*, which contains a perceptive introduction to Keats's 'Ode on Melancholy', pp. 219–21.
59. To Bailey, 18, 22 July 1818, *LJK*, 1, p. 341.
60. Quoted Jackson, p. 84.
61. To Marian Jeffrey, 17, 18 May 1818, *LJK*, 1, p. 287.
62. There is extensive scholarship on Keats's medical training. The most detailed analysis of his time as a medical student is Barnard, '"The busy time", pp. 199–218. There have been other studies on specialist aspects, among them de Almeida, *Romantic Medicine and John Keats*; Goellnicht, *The Poet-Physician: Keats and Medical Science*; Ghosh, *John Keats's Medical Notebooks*. See also R. S. White, 'Like Aesculapius of Old': Keats's Medical Training', 'Keats and the Crisis of Medicine in 1815' and *John Keats, A Literary Life*; Hessell, 'John Keats, the Botanists' Companion'; Ghosh, 'Keats at Guy's Hospital: Moments, Meetings, Choices, and Poems'; Roe, *John Keats: A New Life*; Boyce and Evans, 'The art of medicine: Nothing but flowers'; Evans, 'Poison Wine – John Keats and the Botanic Pharmacy'; and Ruston, 'John Keats, Poet-Physician'.
63. To Reynolds 3 May 1818, *LJK*, p. 277.
64. To Taylor, 24 April 1818,*LJK*, 1, p. 270.
65. See the very thorough account in Holloway, 'The Apothecaries Act, 1815: A Reinterpretation. Part 1. The Origins of the Act', and 'The Apothecaries' Act, 1815: A Reinterpretation. Part 2. The Consequences of the Act'.
66. Porter, *Blood and Guts: A Short History of Medicine*, p. 73.
67. See R. S. White, 'Keats and the Crisis of Medicine in 1815'.
68. Ghosh, 'John Keats's "Guy's Hospital" Poetry', pp. 1–20.
69. R. Campbell, *The London Tradesman*.
70. See Holloway, 'The Apothecaries Act, 1815 . . .'.
71. Rivlin, 'Medical Education', p. 58.
72. For a general historical account, see Porter, *Flesh in the Age of Reason*.
73. Burch, 'The Beauty of Bodysnatching', pp. 43–56, 47.
74. Burch, 'Astley Paston Cooper (1768–1841), anatomist, radical and surgeon'. See also Moore, *The Knife Man: Blood, Body-Snatching and the Birth of Modern Surgery*.
75. 'Aesculapius', *Oracular Communications*.

76. Brown, p. 43.
77. Roe, 'Mr. Keats' in Roe, *John Keats and the Medical Imagination*, pp. 57–72.
78. R. S. White, 'Keats and the Crisis of Medicine in 1815'. See also Hillas Smith, pp. 52–5.
79. Porter, 'The Patient's View: Doing Medical History from Below', p. 193.
80. To the George Keatses, 3 March 1819, *LJK* 2, p. 70.
81. Ziegenhagen, 'Keats, Professional Medicine, and the Two Hyperions'.
82. Pladek, *The Poetics of Palliation*.
83. To George and Tom, 22 December, 1817, *LJK*, 1, p. 192.
84. Bion, p. 31.
85. Sigler, 'Negative Capability in Psychoanalysis: Keats and Retroactive Judgment in Bion, Freud, Lacan and Milner'.
86. Voller, 'Negative Capability: The psychotherapist's X-factor?'; 'Negative Capability'.
87. See also Williams, *The Aesthetic Development: The Poetic Spirit of Psychoanalysis: Essays on Bion, Melzer, Keats*.
88. Cornish, 'Negative Capability and Social Work: Insights from Keats, Bion and Business'.
89. French and Simpson, 'Negative Capability and the Capacity to Think in the Present Moment'.
90. Wilson, p. 18.

Chapter 5

Keats as a Reader of Robert Burton's
The Anatomy of Melancholy

This chapter is something of a leviathan, fittingly so, given the bloated proportions of *The Anatomy of Melancholy*, written by Robert Burton under the pseudonym 'Democritus Junior'. It is difficult to appreciate his distinctive style, reliance on authorities, and characteristic thought processes without quoting at some length, and Keats's markings and annotations on the text are multifarious. An eccentric work which still has a cult following, Burton's gigantic book sounds (and looks, in any of its sundry editions) like a lugubrious and weighty study of antiquarian interest only, but this is not the case at all, as the passages Keats chose to mark, annotate and transcribe fully will, I hope, demonstrate. Despite being full of analysis of serious medical, emotional and psychological matters, and wearying in its copious classical quotations and references, it is also by turns lighthearted, enlightened, witty, and bawdy.

Charles Brown presented Keats with a copy of at least the second volume of the two-volume 1813 edition of *The Anatomy of Melancholy*, dating it by hand '1819'. It seems that after Keats's death Brown reclaimed the book, which was in turn bequeathed to his son and thence passed to Sir Charles Dilke.[1] It is now in the Keats House collection in Hampstead. Brown himself at some stage had marked some passages in the book, but he characteristically used pencil, whereas Keats routinely used ink to mark and annotate his books.

'The Eve of St Agnes' shows traces of Burton's *Anatomy*, which is claimed as a source by biographers and editors. Since Keats was writing this poem between 18 January and 2 February 1819, and since the copy of Burton is dated 1819, it would seem that Brown gave it to Keats in the first two weeks of January.[2] Another possibility is that Keats had begun reading Brown's copy earlier, and that later Brown gave it to him, realising how much his friend was enjoying it. 'The Eve' was revised in September when Keats was beginning to think about compiling his collection. 'La Belle Dame Sans Merci', written on 21 April

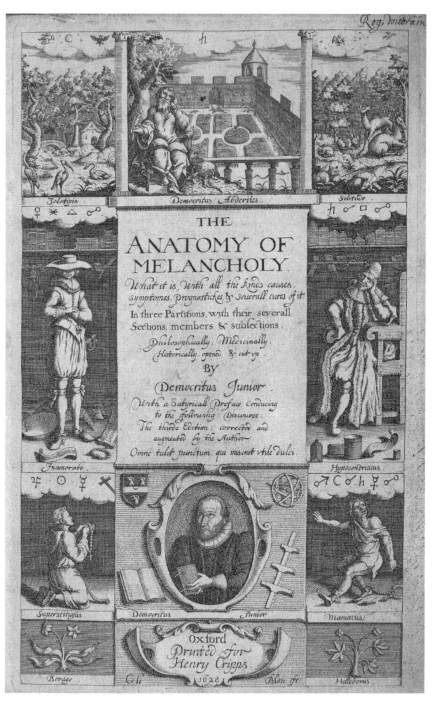

5.1 Title page Robert Burton, *The Anatomy of Melancholy* (1628); British Library, shelfmark C.123.k.281. In the public domain

1819 and published on 10 May 1820, has some clear verbal echoes of Burton, which we shall come to examine below. 'Lamia' was written in June–July, 1819, and Keats in the 1820 volume acknowledges Burton as its major source. Then in September 1819, writing to George and Georgiana Keats (quoted below), Keats speaks of having been 'reading lately' the book, and transcribes a long quotation from Burton, commenting 'I would give my favourite leg to have written this as a speech in a Play'.[3] The evidence seems clear, then, that Keats was given the copy of Burton in early January 1819; was reading, marking, and consulting it right through the year; and that it inevitably had discernible and substantial significance for his own poetry written during that year. However, although his ownership of the book can be dated in this way, it certainly did not inaugurate his interest in melancholy, and it may not have been Keats's first acquaintance with Burton. For example, 'Isabella', written a year earlier in March–April 1818, is one of his most intense and disturbing poems on the subject.

We also know that Keats at one stage owned volume 1, since Brown, in his list of Keats's books, specifies there were two volumes amongst the bequest.[4] Given his obvious enthusiasm for volume 2 it seems almost certain that Keats would have read volume 1 just as closely. At least Robert Gittings tacitly assumes he did, by suggesting some lines in that volume which he suggests are echoed in Keats's poems.[5] Keats's friend Benjamin Haydon, the painter, when he came to sell books in 1823 (after Keats's death) to cover his regular impecunity, included a volume of Burton among them, and one wonders if the volume 1 which Keats had owned ended up in his hands.[6] Keats's informal will, sent to Taylor on August 14, 1820, had concluded with the sentence 'My Chest of Books divide among my friends'.[7]

The 'Hampstead' edition of the Buxton Formans' *The Complete Works of John Keats* transcribed Keats's annotations of Burton and his own, somewhat puzzling, 'index' at the end of the book,[8] but there are also hundreds of underlinings and side-markings which are not reproduced. These are rarely examined and have not been analysed thoroughly in terms of Keats's reading habits and tastes, and his insights into Burton, though Robert Gittings, Janice Sinson, and Aileen Ward have written briefly on ways in which the *Anatomy* may have influenced his own writing. Keats also at some stage acquired an 'abridged', one-volume version of the *Anatomy* (which must have been the 1801 edition since it was not reprinted again until 1824), also listed amongst his legacy of books.[9] His own copy is now lost, but the 1801 abridged version can still be viewed in learned libraries. Its criteria for choosing what to include and exclude seems to be guided by selecting morally improving and religious pieties and excising the more racy and colour-ful elements. Keats no doubt took a dim view of such bowdlerisation, since his manifest interest lies in the frequent scatological and satirical material, as we shall see. However, this short and selective adaptation raises a central point when we go on to look at Keats's markings, since it suggests at the outset that the *Anatomy* is such an extraordinarily roomy and roaming work that entirely different versions of Burton's literary temperament can be discerned and constructed. These range from Lamb's image of 'a man often assoiled by deepest melancholy, and at other times much given to laughing and jesting', to a moralis-ing scholar steeped in serious classical learning, religious issues, and ancient medical practice, through to the relatively conventional piety of a cleric who, in a passage side-marked by Keats, claims little more than 'to collect and glean a few remedies, and comfortable speeches out of our best orators, philosophers, divines, and fathers of the church' (p. 1). The chosen *persona* of the writer, 'Democritus Junior', a 'laugh-ing philosopher', is clearly a mouthpiece for Burton's many-faceted opinions on a bewildering range of subjects.

In the first volume, Burton had itemised causes and symptoms of mel-ancholy as a whole field. The second volume (the one marked by Keats) includes the Second Partition which deals with 'Cure of Melancholy', and the Third Partition on both 'Love-Melancholy' and 'Religious Melancholy' (p. 479). Burton distinguishes himself from other writers, who consider excessive love or religion to be mania or madness, by saying he believes they are melancholy conditions, though he leaves open whether religious melancholy is a subsection of love-melancholy or a 'distinct species' (p. 479). Keats marks each section equally and copiously. Since it is frankly impossible to know or even guess the exact reasons behind Keats's many markings on Burton's *The Anatomy of Melancholy*, I hope what will emerge from this study are patterns of temperamental, philosophical and stylistic affinities, which provide background to interpreting the poems in his own 1820 volume. It is also impossible to deal with all the markings in a chapter, since there are so many of them, so my account will be highly selective, in the hope that general points will emerge. To anticipate a conclusion, just as Burton uses melancholy as a hook upon which to hang a bewilderingly diverse set of subjects and moods, so Keats, exercising his intuitively enquiring temperament and immersive reading habit with pen in hand, manages to appreciate the eclecticism of Burton's approach, and to foreground many of the stylistic and tonal modulations in *The Anatomy*, as well as reflecting its extraordinarily wide-ranging study of melancholy. In general terms, the following areas emerge as of interest to Keats:

1. Varieties of melancholy, especially in relation to love.
2. Reading as a poet: stylistic and thematic aspects.
3. Personal, biographical or 'life' preoccupations of Keats (such as health and weather).
4. Burton as 'the human friend the philosopher': memorable expressions of thought and ideas.
5. Storytelling and anecdotes.
6. Humour and bawdy.
7. Epigrammatical phrases, *sententiae*.
8. Reading as a trained surgeon-apothecary: medical references.
9. Keats's 'Index' at the end of the volume, which rather mysteriously itemises sections of interest to him.

However, since these areas overlap so much it is unnecessary to keep them apart in our analysis, and besides, several can be exemplified in individual quotations, so examples will be used to illustrate various aspects of Keats's readings. In particular, I limit my coverage to some leading issues which seem of relevance to Keats's 1820 volume: medical and poetic content, the subject of love, and some speculations about Keats's unique 'index' of certain incidents, which he lists at the end of his copy of the *Anatomy*. In transcribing the markings, I use italics to indicate where Keats side-marks (not distinguishing whether single, double, broken, or unbroken), and underline what he underlines. Page numbers in my text refer to Keats's 1813 edition, and where a passage appears in the first volume, I indicate its place in Burton's book.

The thematic concentration on different typologies of melancholy, both literary and medical in origin, frame Keats's 1820 collection, I argue, with his own condensed, poetic 'anatomy of melancholy' for his own age. Moreover, at the level of detail, reading adjacent poems with an eye to Burton's influence and in the order Keats planned, reveals many verbal, imagistic and rhythmical 'chimes' and parallels explored in Chapter 6. Keats's evidently intense reading of Burton's book during the period when he was writing and selecting the poems for his own volume, may have enabled him to bring to light the subject he himself had been constantly living, thinking and writing about, the complex condition of melancholy in its historical, literary, and personal contexts.

Despite its claim to be based on a methodical analytical system indicated in the meticulous, taxonomically arranged table of contents or 'Synopsis', Robert Burton's *The Anatomy of Melancholy* is constantly digressive, anecdotal, opinionated and far from systematic, proceeding instead in a subjectively driven stream of consciousness, readily admitted by Burton himself:

'tis not my study or intent to compose neatly, which an orator requires, but to express myself readily and plainly as it happens. So that as a river runs sometimes precipitate and swift, then dull and slow; now direct, then *per ambages*, now deep, then shallow; now muddy, then clear; now broad, then narrow; doth my style flow: now serious, then light; now comical, then satirical; now more elaborate, then remiss, as the present subject required, or as at that time I was affected. And if thou vouchsafe to read this treatise, it shall seem no otherwise to thee, than the way to an ordinary traveller, sometimes fair, sometimes foul; here champaign, there enclosed; barren, in one place, better soil in another: by woods, groves, hills, dales, plains, &c. I shall lead thee *per ardua montium, et lubrica vallum, et roscida cespitum, et glebosa camporum* [through heights of mountains, and the slippery embankment, and the dew-wet ground, and clods of the valleys], through variety of objects, that which thou shalt like and surely dislike.

[*Anatomy*, 1,18,6–12][10]

Such descriptions by Burton of his own style undoubtedly reflect *The Anatomy of Melancholy*'s multifaceted and quirky aspects which appealed to Keats, whose own unique, irrepressible sense of humour, 'now serious, then light; now comical, then satirical', often reframing grim situations with word-play, and droll mockery, corresponds to similar qualities in Burton. We detect a stylistic resemblance in Keats's description to Reynolds of his own epistolary composition as 'like a Rat-trap', similarly associative and emotionally variegated, and held together by free-wheeling thought processes and subjectivity of personality rather than logic: 'for by merely touching the spring delicately and etherially, the rough-edged will fly immediately into a proper compactness, and thus you may make a good wholesome loaf, with your own leven in it, of my fragments . . . '.[11] This may also offer us a clue into Keats's process of reading books such as Burton's. In marking and annotating 'fragments' and providing his own personal 'leven' of opinions, he is constructing the text to reflect a 'compactness' reflecting his own priorities. By following his markings on his copy of the *Anatomy* we can see what he appreciated in a writer who in some ways was a kindred spirit. In the final chapter of this book we shall see some specific examples of Keats using the *Anatomy* as inspiration for his poetry, but in this chapter I shall suggest some of the aspects of his reading practices which we can deduce from his markings and annotations, and seek to understand what kinds of things strike the poet as interesting and potentially useful for his own work.

Responsive Reading

The account that follows relies methodologically on reader-response criticism (sometimes known as reader-centred theory)[12] in two senses: I am 'reading' Keats's markings as he reads Burton's text. Such an approach unashamedly involves subjective judgment and it is not so much a 'theory' as a set of assumptions like these:

> A text only becomes meaningful when it is read, when a reader interacts with the words on the page to produce meaning. What we call reading is an active participation on the part of the reader to construct meaning from a piece of writing . . . A text is the temporal experience of reading which actualizes meaning, the experience of which is specific to each individual reader.[13]

Reader-response as a 'theory' had a vigorous and promising inauguration in the works of Wolfgang Iser, Norman Holland, Hans Robert Jauss and others in the 1970s and '80s.[14] Roland Barthes's provocative phrase, 'the death of the author' was intended to refocus attention on the text irrespective of authorial intentions, but it also encapsulated one part of the reader-response approach, which proclaimed the birth of the reader as a consequence of believing in the plural potential of a text to stimulate diverse readings.[15] It is analogous to reception theory in performance and media studies, where an audience's reactions are analysed in relation to the object of their attention, like going to the theatre to observe the audience as much as the play. In this context, audiences may be viewed as interpretive communities, responding both as collective entities and as individuals. In reader-response criticism the equivalent might be described as 'reading the reader' interrelating with the text, acknowledging the individuality of the reader recording a uniquely creative reading process. In this sense a reader's personality, readerly intentions, range of interests acquired through cultural conditioning and experience, and prior knowledge, are all actively engaged in reading, an act of constructing the content of the text in a unique way on each occasion. Emotions are involved as well, and since reading is a relational experience, a reader may sympathetically identify with the text (enjoy it, become engrossed) or resist its assumptions (become angry, irritated or bored), or anything in between.[16] It may change his or her attitudes, or have no effect. A further implication is that even the same individual reader will make different readings, and construct different texts, on each occasion, since she or he is constantly in a state of change; books that absorbed and delighted a person in childhood may be encountered with indifference or even abhorrence as an adult. In this sense texts are not fixed or unchanging, and nor are readers.

In fact, there is good reason to credit Keats himself with the seeds for this approach. Cassandra Falkes uses the phrase 'Negatively Capable Reading' to 'define the kind of knowledge one gains from literature'.[17] She likens the 'ineffable, experiential knowledge' acquired through reading to Keats's 'negative Capability' as the thought processes of one who 'is capable of being in uncertainties, Mysteries, doubts, without any irritable reaching after fact & reason'.[18] Keats was speaking of writing, especially that of Shakespeare, but the idea can be applied just as fruitfully to reading. Cowden Clarke recalled that Keats 'devoured rather than read' books borrowed from the school library. Whether he was 'burning' through *King Lear* or reading *The Faerie Queene*, in Clarke's words, 'as a young horse would through a spring meadow – ramping!'.[19] In the present context, this is made doubly complex by the fact that we are reading one book (Burton's) through the eyes of another reader (Keats), and such an exercise requires not only a high tolerance for uncertainty but also a suspension of final judgments. We simply cannot know what was exactly in Keats's mind when he marked a passage in Burton's *Anatomy*, but we can at least assume he regarded it as in some way noteworthy, important, or useful to him. Here I hope to illustrate some of the *kinds* of words and passages that attracted him, but will try not to impose too rigid an explanation for *why* he took up his pen.[20] The enterprise seems justified as an exploration of the creative process of reading and writing practised by Keats, as an activity along a continuum running from open-minded empiricism to the self-assertion of poetic composition.

Beth Lau in *Keats's Paradise Lost* provides an exemplary description of what we might look for when inspecting Keats's markings and annotations of another text which was supremely important to him:

> At the least, discovering recurring themes and patterns in Keats's *Paradise Lost* marginalia extends our awareness of how pervasive these tendencies and preoccupations were in the poet's outlook and sharpens our understanding of Keats's handling of the same topics and techniques in his own work. Certainly the marginalia can yield a number of insights into Keats's personality and habits of mind, into the nature of Milton's impact on Keats, and into the dynamics of literary influence and the reading process.[21]

Referring to the precedent of Spurgeon's *Keats's Shakespeare: A Descriptive Study*,[22] Lau adopts the ideal procedure of supplying the evidence by transcribing the markings and annotations on Keats's *Paradise Lost*, so that her readers can make up their own minds. However, in the case of his copious markings of Burton, there are so many that this is impossible without overbalancing the proportions of this book (or without supplying another hefty volume). Quite apart from the sheer quantity of Keats's detailed markings, there are whole pages at a time which are side-marked. There are hundreds of markings, incorporating thousands of words, and surplus to requirements in this book which is offered as a work of criticism rather than transcription. Without claiming expertise as a mind-reader, I hope instead to extrapolate some general conclusions that seem to emerge from 'reading over Keats's shoulder' as he reads, pen in hand. It is in some ways the very *ad hoc* randomness of the evidence which is at least part of the point, reflecting both Burton's omnivorous curiosity and willingness to be diverted by detail, as Keats's desire 'to let the mind be a thoroughfare for all thoughts'.[23] The 'camelion Poet' is equally a chameleon reader:

> What shocks the virtuous philosop[h]er, delights the camelion Poet. It does no harm from its relish of the dark side of things any more than from its taste for the bright one; because they both end in speculation.[24]

In this sense, the ideal reader encounters the ideal text, since Burton is by turns both a judgmental 'virtuous philosopher' and a writer with a poet's imagination, 'every thing and nothing', enjoying 'light and shade', demonstrating an empirical open-mindedness replicated in Keats as reader.

Fortuitously, we have a uniquely direct comparison which might elegantly demonstrate how different can be the personal and idiosyncratic habits of selection and reading processes practised by individual readers, even ones apparently with generally compatible literary interests. The exact same text of volume 2 of Burton's *Anatomy* printed in 1813, now in the Bodleian Library at Oxford,[25] according to the signature on the title page, was 'George Taylor's'. He clearly read every page very attentively and the frequent markings presumably made by him use the same style of handwriting in pen and ink as Keats. At the very least this copy shows similar manual habits of readers of the time in annotating books. Taylor uses roughly the same combination of underlining, side-marking and marginal notes, whose position in the text he indicates by a cross (x or +), though unlike Keats he frequently uses 'NB' to call attention to some detail, and he sometimes employs dotted lines in his side-markings. One of his annotations refers to using horses to deliver mail in 'Nov. 1821', which might date his reading (p. 431) and establish Taylor's reading as contemporary with Keats's in 1819. We can gauge from the markings a lot of Taylor's learned and even pedantic temperament. He is clearly at least as well read as Keats, able to spot and identify (often even citing page number) literary quotations and allusions to a range of works and writers particularly from the eighteenth century, such as 'x Tristram Shandy Vol. 5. (Ch. 3ᵈ. Ed. 1803)' (on Burton's text p. 58), Cowley (pp. 365 and 505), Oldham (p. 375), Livy (p. 395), Swift (p. 456), Cornelius Tacitus (the reference attributed to 'Joe Miller' whose *Joe Miller's Jest Book, or, the Wit's Vade-Mecum* was published first in 1739 and reprinted several times) (p. 464), 'Hobbes, Leviathan preface' (p. 554), Shakespeare, in a quotation as esoteric as an Old Lady in *Henry 8*, no less (p. 566), and others less well known.

The point that Taylor notes Sterne's indebtedness to Burton is important here, since Keats also notices in Burton's text anticipations of Sterne's *Tristram Shandy*. Both he and Taylor recognised a controversy that still rages among scholars, whether Sterne plagiarises or creatively borrows from Burton.[26] Sterne's extensive habit of quoting from Burton without attribution was exposed in Keats's time by another man of letters and self-confessed 'bibliomania' enthusiast who was also a qualified, publishing physician, John Ferriar of Manchester. In his book *Illustrations of Sterne* (1798), Ferriar voluminously documents many of the very close borrowings.[27] Being equally fond of both books, he suggests that the quotations are often purposeful in characterising Mr Shandy, who, 'with all the stains and mouldiness of the last century about him, I am now convinced that most of the singularities of that character were drawn from the perusal of Burton' (p. 57). So, in a sense, Keats would have read exactly the same passages in both Sterne and Burton – and if he had read Ferriar's book (not entirely unlikely) he would have found them quoted yet a third time. This provides another possible answer to the open question, whether Keats had read the first volume of Burton's *Anatomy*. Even if he had not, Sterne provided him with some passages, which Ferriar identified from Burton's Volume 1. Here is a nice example which Keats, as erstwhile apothecary, would surely have found irresistible, from Burton's Introduction, as his persona describes his method of composition, some of which is repeated in *Tristram Shandy* (Book V, Chapter 1):

> As apothecaries we make new mixtures everyday, pour out of one vessel into another; and as those old Romans robbed all the cities of the world, to set out their bad-sited Rome, we skim off the cream of other men's wits, pick the choice flowers of their tilled gardens to set out our own sterile plots . . . A fault that every writer finds, as I do now, and yet faulty themselves, *Trium literarum homines*, all thieves; they pilfer out of old writers to stuff up their new comments, scrape Ennius' dunghills, and out of Democritus' pit, as I have done. ('Democritus Junior to the Reader')

Both books were amongst Keats's favourites, and Herbert Read detected a temperamental affinity between Sterne and Keats:

> We know that Keats was familiar with *Tristram Shandy*, and it may be that his notion of *Negative Capability* ... owes something to Sterne's character of Yorick – in any case, Sterne was certainly also 'a man capable of being in uncertainties, Mysteries, doubts'.[28]

Much the same could be said of Burton. Despite his best endeavours to find answers for everything, the sheer eclecticism builds up the opposite impression, of one revelling in contradictions and uncertainty.

Taylor assiduously reaches for books, whether from his shelves or found in a well-stocked library, to track down exact references for some Latin translations even in Burton's footnotes, such as ones from Virgil (p. 199) and Tacitus (p. 479). He queries of a couplet in English whether 'Etherege borrowed this?' (p. 377) and points out the odd misprint or misquotation in the *Anatomy* (for example p. 189). Building on Burton's own practice, he is prone to adding other ancient sources, quoting in Greek himself (p. 389), and he fastidiously adds occasional references even in the index. He shows occasional knowledge of medical practice, noting details such as trepanning the skull 'to let out the fuliginous vapours' in Burton's phrase, 'bad spirit' in Taylor's (p. 124). Like Keats, his eye and pen sometimes alight on unusual, now obsolete words like 'tenterbellies' (p. 352) for 'those who distend their bellies; gluttons'.[29]

Taylor's reading is as animated, active, interrogative and exclamatory as we shall find Keats's to be, and yet the two readers have only a limited percentage of marked passages in common, indicating that they are choosing different areas of interest to highlight in the text. Taylor reveals himself as classically trained in Greek and Latin, almost certainly to university level, and perhaps even a don like Burton himself with access to a scholarly library. Clearly he was philologically inclined, and well read in eighteenth century English literature and drama, but seemingly without Keats's characteristic sense of fun.[30] He lacks the kind of annotations given by Keats, who constantly jots brief expressions of appreciation, such as single exclamation marks and words like 'Pshaw!' (p. 367), 'good –' (p. 385), 'mum' (p. 401), 'aye – aye' (p. 417), 'extraordinary' (p. 507), 'good' (p. 510). Beside Burton's coinage 'pseudo-martyrs' (p. 510), Keats wrote 'The most biggotted [sic] word ever met with – '. Beside Burton's 'be thou still Caius, I'll be Caia', Keats jots 'Jack and Jill', answering humour with humour, and when Burton mentions 'Italian blaspheming, Spanish renouncing' Keats writes 'O that he had gone through all the nations!'. In terms of reader-response theory Keats constructs Burton very differently from

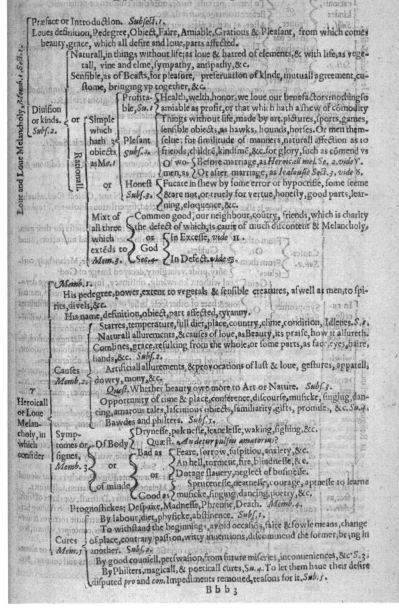

ANALYSIS OF THE
THIRD PARTITION.

Loue and Loue Melancholy, Memb.1,Sect.1.

Præface or Introduction. *Subsect.1.*

Loues definition, Pedegree, Obiect, Faire, Amiable, Gratious & Pleasant, from which comes beauty, grace, which all desire and loue, parts affected.

Naturall, in things without life; as loue & hatred of elements, & with life, as vegetall, vine and elme, sympathy, antipathy, &c.

Sensible, as of Beasts, for pleasure, preseruation of kinde, mutuall agreement, custome, bringing vp together, &c.

Diuision or kinds. *Subs.2.* — or — Rationall. — Simple which hath 3 obiects, as Me.1

Profitable, *Su.1* — Health, welth, honor, we loue our benefactors: nothing so amiable as profit, or that which hath a shew of comodity

Plesant *subs.2.* — Things without life, made by art, pictures, sports, games, sensible obiects, as hawks, hounds, horses. Or men themselue: for similitude of manners, naturall affection as to friends, childre, kindsme, &c. for glory, such as comend vs

Honest *Subs.3.* — Of wo- { Before marriage, as Heroicall mel. Se. 2. vide Y. men, as { Or after marriage, as Iealousie Sect. 3. vide δ.

Fucate in shew by some error or hypocrisie, some seeme & are not, or truely for vertue, honesty, good parts, learning, eloquence, &c.

Mixt of all three which extēds to God *Mem.3.* — Common good, our neighbour, coutry, friends, which is charity the defect of which, is cause of much discontent & Melancholy,

or { In Excesse, vide II.
God *Sect.4.* { In Defect. vide ꝗ.

Heroicall or Loue Melancholy, in which consider

Memb.1.

His pedegree, power, extent to vegetals & sensible creatures, aswell as men, to spirits, diuels, &c.

His name, definition, obiect, part affected, tyranny.

Causes *Memb.2.* —

Starres, temperature, full diet, place, country, clime, condition, Idlenes. *S.1.*

Naturall allurements, & causes of loue, as Beauty, its praise, how it assureth. Comlines, grace, resulting from the whole, or some parts, as face, eyes, haire, hands, &c. *Subf.2.*

Artificiall allurements, & prouocations of lust & loue, gestures, apparell, dowry, mony, &c.

Quæst. Whether beauty owe more to Art or Nature. *Subf.3.*

Opportunity of time & place, conference, discourse, musicke, singing, dancing, amarous tales, lasciuious obiects, familiarity, gifts, promise, &c. *Su.4.*

Bawdes and philters. *Subf.5.*

Symptomes or signes, *Memb.3.*

Of Body {
Drynesse, pakenesse, leanelesse, waking, sighing, &c.

Quæst. An detur pulsus amatorius?

Bad as { Feare, sorrow, suspition, anxiety, &c. An hell, torment, fire, blindnesse, &c.

or { Dotage slauery, neglect of businesse.

of minde {
Good as { Sprucenesse, neatnesse, courage, aptnesse to learne musicke, singing, dancing, poetry, &c.

Prognostickes; Despaire, Madnesse, Phrensie, Death. *Memb.4.*

Cures *Mem.5.* —

By labour, diet, physicke, abstinence. *Subf.1.*

To withstand the beginning, auoid occasion, faire & fowle means, change of place, contrary passion, witty inuentions, discommend the former, bring in another. *Subf.2.*

By good counsell, perswasion, from future miseries, inconueniences, &c. *S.3.*

By Philters, magicall, & poeticall cures, *Su.4.* To let them haue their desire disputed pro and con. Impediments remoued, reasons for it. *Subf.5.*

5.2 Burton on Love, 'Analysis of the Third Partition', Robert Burton, *The Anatomy of Melancholy* (1628); British Library, shelfmark C.123.k.281 (15). In the public domain.

George Taylor's scholarly, learned, literary, and apparently humourless responses. Keats's primary interest was also, like Taylor's, literary (if somewhat less pedantic) and even philological, since he often marks Latin quotations, no doubt building upon or testing out his knowledge gleaned from his school prize for translating Virgil. However, he is also clearly interested in the substantive subject of melancholy from a medical and curative perspective, and his markings reveal alert interests as diverse and scattered as Burton's own. The comparison between Taylor's and Keats's markings reveals quite different personalities and interests. Other annotated copies of the *Anatomy* from the nineteenth century are appearing in auctions, making it, among other things, a significant document in the history of reading.[31]

Keats as a Reader of Burton's *Anatomy of Melancholy*

In a letter he wrote to George and Georgiana Keats, 17–27 September 1819, Keats quotes from Burton at some length:

I have been reading lately Burton's Anatomy of Melancholy; and I think you will be very much amused with a page I here coppy for you. I call it a Feu de joie round the batteries of Fort S[t] Hyphen-de-Phrase on the birthday of the Digamma. The whole alphabet was drawn up in a Phalanx on the cover of an old Dictionary. Band playing "Amo, Amas &c" "Every Lover admires his Mistress, though she be very deformed of herself, ill-favoured, wrinkled, pimpled, pale, red, yellow, tann'd, tallow-fac'd, have a swoln juglers platter face, or a thin, lean, chitty face, have clouds in her face, be crooked, dry, bald, goggle-eyed, blear-eyed or with staring eyes, she looks like a squis'd cat, hold her head still awry, heavy, dull, hollow-eyed, black or yellow about the eyes, or squint-eyed, sparrow-mouth'd, Persean hook-nosed, have a sharp fox nose, a red nose, China flat, great nose, nare simo patuloque, a nose like a promontory, gubber-tush'd, rotten teeth, black, uneven, brown teeth, beetle brow'd, a witches beard, her breath stink all over the room, her nose drop winter and summer, with a Bavarian poke under her chin, a sharp chin, lave-eared, with a long crane's neck, which stands awry too, pendulis mammis her dugs like two double jugs, or else no dugs in the other extream, bloody-falln fingers, she have filthy, long unpaired nails, scabbed hands or wrists, a tan'd skin, a rotton carcass, crooked back, she stoops, is lame, splea footed, as slender in the middle as a cow in the wast, gowty legs, her ankles hang over her shooes, her feet stink, she breed lice, a meer changeling, a very monster, an aufe imperfect, her whole complexion savors, an harsh voice, incondite gesture, vile gate, a vast virago, or an ugly tit, a slug, a fat fustilugs, a trusse, a long lean rawbone, a Skeleton, a Sneaker (si qua latent meliora puta), and to thy Judgement looks like a mard in a Lanthorn, whom thou couldst not fancy for a world, but hatest, loathest, and wouldst have spit in her face, or blow thy nose in her bosom, remedium amoris to another man, a dowdy, a Slut, a scold, a nasty rank, rammy, filthy, beastly quean, dishonest per adventure, obscene, base, beggarly, rude, foolish, untaught – peevish, Irus' daughter, Thersites' sister, Grobians' Scholler; if he love her once, he admires her for all this, he takes no notice of any such errors, or imperfections of boddy or mind –" There's a dose for you – fine!! I would give my favourite leg to have written this as a speech in a Play: with what effect could Matthews pop-gun it at the pit! This I think will amuse you more than so much Poetry. Of that I do not like to copy any as I am affraid it is too mal apropos for you at present – and yet I will send you some – for by the time you receive it things in England may have taken a different turn.[32]

Charles Mathews was a popular comic actor and impressionist, a friend of Hunt and of Dickens.[33] Beside the passage in Burton, Keats annotates with the words that he includes in the letter to introduce the quotation:

Feu de Joi round the Batteries of Fort St. Hyphen de Phrase – on the Birthday of the Digamma. The whole alphabet was drawn up into a Phalanx on the cover of an old Dictionary – Band playing 'amo amas I lov'd a Lass'.

Keats signals that he is playing with language, inspired by Burton's own neologisms and linguistic fertility. *Feu de joie* ('fire of joy') is French for either bonfire or armed salute,[34] and Keats is appreciating the passage at a verbal level as an explosion of colourful words and syntax, noting with infectious delight hyphens ('tallow-fac'd', 'goggle-eyed', 'gubber-tush'd', 'bloody-fall'n'), riotous phrases ('a squis'd cat', 'a nasty rank, rammy, filthy, beastly quean'), and employing a uniquely Burtonian 'Dictionary' ('fustilugs'). 'Digamma' is a Greek consonant for 'double-gamma', standing for the letter 'waw' or the number 6, but Keats is no doubt using it without precision and simply emphasising his level of interest as mainly focused on language. There is certainly much to catch his eye in Burton's linguistic 'fireworks'.

However, the meaning too reflects sentiments that Burton regularly reiterates and Keats often marks, especially the rhetoric of satirical disgust and bodily repulsion, more often than not is attached to women, and amplified with unpleasant expressions of misogyny. The attitude to women is (reprehensibly) a constant Burtonian refrain which arouses him to such verbal flights of invective. As a cloistered celibate at Oxford it is an open question how many women he actually observed in his day-to-day living. He is also sarcastic about the bodily infirmities of the elderly, men and women alike. The sardonic sentiment which the context of the quotation implies about love is typical of Burton, and again attracts Keats's attention. On the page Keats is transcribing (p. 314), Burton improvises on a theme which he repeats many times, the discrepancy between the lover's perception and the object of love: 'love

is blind, as the saying is, Cupid's blind, and so are all his followers . . .
Quisquis amat ranam, ranam putat esse Dianam' (anyone who loves a
frog thinks that frog to be Diana)'. In his copy of Burton, Keats carefully
underlined and side-marked Burton's passage down to '<u>imperfections
of body and mind</u>', and then he underlines another phrase in the next
sentence:

> O that he had but the wealth and treasure of both the Indies to endow her
> with, a carrack of diamonds, a chain of pearl, a cascanet of jewels, <u>a pair of
> calf skin gloves of four-pence a pair were fitter</u>), or some such toy, to send
> her for a token . . .

The satirical, debunking mode demonstrated here is typical of Burton,
and evidently appealed to Keats. The example shows him reading Burton
with interactive and alert excitement, and an exhilarated admiration
for the self-generating potency of colourful language. He envisages the
passage as ripe for recitation on the stage. The content and tones are also
typical of what Keats notices time and again. However, the main point
Burton is making, and which Keats is surely noticing, is the blindness of
all lovers, men and women, to the human imperfections of their object
of adoration. The jaundiced attitude to women in particular will be
observed later when we come to look in detail at 'Lamia'.

The critics who have studied the markings and marginalia, namely
Robert Gittings, Janice Sinson and Aileen Ward, agree on these points
(with slight differences in dating), but they disagree about how much it
influenced Keats's own poetry. Gittings in *The Living Year*, and Janice
Sinson in *John Keats and the Anatomy of Melancholy*, claim a lot: Ward
is more cautious and limited. In two statements Ward suggests how she
sees the nature of some of Keats's interests. She observes without comment
that his markings show Keats was most engaged with the sections on
medicinal plants, and on love.[35] On the former, it is not surprising that
Keats was especially interested in botany since the evidence suggests this
was by far his favourite branch of medicine at Guy's. Excursions to the
Apothecaries Garden (now the Chelsea Physic Garden) and Hampstead
Heath and the garden of his teacher, William Salisbury, seem to have
been amongst his most enjoyable hours in studying medicine.[36] There is
no evidence he was actually enrolled in the botany course, but it seems
overwhelmingly likely he attended.[37] This conclusion is reinforced by
the little sketches he did of plants while he was taking notes at an
anatomy lecture, and he may well have been carrying his lecture booklet
on such a visit and used the space in the margin to sketch what he saw.
The image is generally interpreted (following the opinion of his fellow
student and flat-mate, Henry Stephens) as showing Keats's boredom in

the lecture theatre as he drifts into a fantasy world of poetry, but it seems just as likely his mind is on the next or previous botany lecture.[38] On love, Ward interprets his interest as purely personal and biographical, whereas, as Gittings shows, a lot of nonspecific but important material about love in Burton points towards the poems. More recently, Andrew Motion has concluded that Keats 'used the Anatomy as a highly selective kind of diary – a private and often extremely bilious grumble-book', annotated with remarks that are 'self-goading or self-lacerating', in particular regarding women and marriage.[39]

Ward concludes further that '*The Anatomy of Melancholy* was important to Keats not for its style but for its ideas'.[40] This seems only half-right since it seems more accurate to say that Keats appreciated *both* style and ideas. However, Ward again veers away from the creative relevance of this perception by adding that the interest was 'a personal and private one'. She does not mention that it is likely that one important 'idea' which drew him to Burton was a professional interest in the history of melancholy itself as a medical condition, as the field had stood in the literary period which he most loved, the Renaissance. Given that nowadays we think of Burton's analyses as 'literature' and as a curiosity, rather than making claims to scholarship, we forget its intention and reception, as a compendious cataloguing based on humoural medicine which was not quite dead in Keats's time in university learning, local medical practices, and in poetry. The subtitle of Burton's book, wittily claiming that its subject is '*Philosophically, Medicinally, Historically, OPENED AND CUT UP*', might have struck Keats as reminiscent of his earlier anatomy classes. Among other things, it was intended as a medical textbook of an exhaustive kind, as J. B. Bamborough summarises:

> Having taken Melancholy as his subject, Burton appears, as a true scholar, to have decided to exhaust the topic, to include all its ramifications and to cite every authority – to produce 'the last word' . . . 'Anatomies' were something of a vogue in the latter part of the sixteenth century. The name implied an attempt to get to the bottom of things and reveal everything fully and methodically.[41]

Keats Reading as a Trained Apothecary: Medical References

Amongst other things, Burton envisaged his *Anatomy* as a medical textbook. Body, mind, emotions and the soul were considered intimately interconnected, so that imbalance in the body caused, or was caused by, imbalance in the mind. In Burton's list of the types of melancholy, we find a range of mental states, from depression, sorrow, lasciviousness, anxiety, terror and anger, through to ecstasy, mania and suicidal thoughts. Even worthy pursuits could lead to melancholy if indulged to excess, like 'love of learning . . . the misery of scholars' and poets – 'why the Muses are melancholy' (Table of Contents). Extreme religious faith or overrationality could lead respectively to the zealot's or philosopher's melancholy, while different kinds of love could also be pathologised in their more overwhelming states. Poets and artists were especially prone to a 'saturnine' form of melancholy which drove them to create imaginative worlds. Symptoms, causes, and remedies were manifold, and in Burton's encyclopaedic account, fascinating. Vestiges of humoural learning survived into Keats's time, such as medical botany and some dietary prescriptions – and after all, he himself during his own illnesses chose regular bloodletting, the most ancient of all 'cures' based on humoural medicine. However, by 1820 Burton's work was read, if at all, mainly by literary figures or antiquarians. For Keats, however, it was evidently much more. He likens himself to Shakespeare's Jaques in *As You Like It* who 'can suck melancholy out of song as a weasel sucks eggs' (2.5.11–12), mentioning in a letter 'I could always find an eggshell for melancholy'.[42] The same could certainly be said for Burton.

The Renaissance was an age of 'anatomies'; of looking beneath the surface by peeling away layers of literal or metaphorical skin. John Donne wrote *The First Anniversary: An Anatomy of the World* in 1611, and William Harvey was physician to James I when he 'anatomised' the circulation of blood, much to the horror of his conservative medical colleagues. The word was used in titles of books ranging in subjects from medicine and religion to politics, including issues like *Anatomy of Infidelity, Anatomy of Independence* and *The Writing Schoolmaster, or The Anatomy of Fair Writing*. By Keats's time, even if the doctrine of humours was no longer uncritically accepted yet some aspects of the older approach were still visible in medical practice. Aileen Ward notes the way Keats marks passages on the importance of climate on health, which was something of a personal obsession for him in terms of his own welfare, and also something that could contribute to atmosphere in many of his poems, including 'The Eve of St Agnes', 'Ode to Psyche', 'To Autumn', 'La Belle Dame' and others, where weather is central.[43] Shahidha Bari has written on the weather and seasonal change in Keats as amounting to a philosophy of phenomenalism,[44] but its origins lie in his acute sensitivity to climatic conditions affecting his medical concerns.

Herbal remedies interest him as part of the apothecary's learning.

Amongst Burton's 'purging simples' to cure 'head melancholy', Keats side-marks,

> 'White hellebore, which some call sneezing-powder': *Christophorus a Vega, lib. 3. c. 41, is of the same opinion, that it may be lawfully given; and our country gentlewomen find it by their common practice, that there is no such great danger in it. Dr. Turner, speaking of this plant in his Herbal, telleth us, that in his time it was an ordinary receipt among good wives, to give hellebore in powder to ii^d weight, and he is not much against it. But they do commonly exceed, for who so bold as blind Bayard, and prescribe it by pennyworths, and such irrational ways, as I have heard myself market folks ask for it in an apothecary's shop: but with what success God knows; they smart often for their rash boldness and folly, break a vein, make their eyes ready to start out of their heads, or kill themselves.* So that the fault is not in the physic, but in the rude and indiscreet handling of it. (p. 107)

Burton refers several times to hellebore, and in Murray's *Materia Medica* (1810), which Keats would have known in his medical training, black hellebore is described as a 'violent' and dangerous cathartic administered in diluted 'watery extract' for 'mania and melancholy, in which diseases it was highly celebrated by the ancients'.[45] Keats had encountered hellebore in botany classes at the Apothecaries Garden, no doubt in both its black and its white varieties; the former, according to Culpepper and Gerard, being 'very effectual against all melancholy diseases'. In addition, as de Almeida notes, the lecturers at Guy's during his time, Babington and Curry, included hellebore amongst remedies for insanity.[46] Keats had already referred to it in the valentine verse letter (sent on George's behalf) to Mary Frogley ('Hadst thou lived in days of old'), written while still a student at Guy's (14 February, 1816), likening Mary's hair to 'many graceful bends: | As the leaves of hellebore | Turn to whence they sprung before . . .'. Burton's passage as a whole demonstrates his own style and personality and reflects social realities of his time, warning that untrained overdoses and 'such irrational ways, as I have heard myself market folks ask for it in an apothecary's shop' can just as easily kill as cure a patient. Tobacco was considered to be another plant which could be both dangerous, and remedial, and Keats places double marking down the side of the passage which both extols and condemns it in Burton's judiciously double vision:

> *Tobacco, divine, rare, superexcellent tobacco, which goes far beyond all the panaceas, potable gold, and philosopher's stones, a sovereign remedy to all diseases. A good vomit, I confess, a virtuous herb, if it be well qualified, opportunely taken, and medicinally used; but as it is commonly abused by most men, which take it as tinkers do ale, 'tis a plague, a mischief, a violent purger of goods, lands, health, hellish, devilish and damned tobacco, the ruin and overthrow of body and soul.* (p. 109)

On alcohol, Burton agrees with the intriguing advice to '*him that is troubled in mind, or melancholy, not to drink only, but now and then to be drunk: excellent good physic it is for this and many other diseases*' (p. 128); though with the caveat, '*Woe be to him that makes his neighbour drunk, shameful spewing shall be upon his glory*' (p. 129). The appeal of this to Keats no doubt was more to his sense of humour than a useful remedial tip. Likewise, Keats shows interest in Burton's recommendations to use precious stones as 'so many several medicines against melancholy, sorrow, fear, dullness, and the like' (p. 97), continuing '"*almost all jewels and precious stones have excellent virtues*" *to pacify the affections of the mind, for which cause rich men so much covet to have them*' (p. 99). Keats sees something like *Tristram Shandy* in this reasoning, and his annotation ends on a wry joke:

> This list of precious stones and their virtues is very curious – it is certainly a slight touch of 'my uncle Toby' because in looking onwards I do not find the *counter-snarle*. Precious stones are certainly a remedy against Melancholy: a valuable diamond would effectually cure mine.

The 'counter-snarle' he expects may refer to Burton's more characteristic way of reasoning, weighing up 'on the one hand this, on the other hand that' approach evident in his words on hellebore, tobacco, and alcohol.

By underlining, Keats pays attention to Burton's sometimes critical view of professional medical practice, which shows awareness of the possibility of charlatans claiming to be physicians:

> '*tis a corrupt trade, no science, art, no profession; the beginning, practice, and progress of it, all is naught, full of imposture, uncertainty, and doth generally more harm than good.* <u>The divell himself was the first inventor of it</u>: *Inventum est medicina meum* [medicine was my invention], *said Apollo,* <u>and what was Apollo, but the divell?</u> *The Greeks first made an art of it, and they were all deluded by Apollo's sons, priests, oracles.* (p. 87)

Keats several times in his poetry associates Apollo benignly with both medicine and poetry, but the distinction drawn by Moneta in *The Fall of Hyperion* – that there are useful and useless poets – would also, in Burton's view, be applied to physicians. Similarly, surgeons and apothecaries, the two professions in which Keats's training was most comprehensive, are not spared the lash of Burton's criticism of physicians, and nor do they escape Keats's attention:

> But it is their ignorance that doth more harm than rashness, their art is wholly conjectural, if it be an art, uncertain, imperfect, and got by killing of men, they are a kind of butchers, leeches, men-slayers; surgeons and apothecaries especially, that are indeed the physicians' hangman, carnifices [butchers],

and common executioners; though to say truth, physicians themselves come not far behind; for according to that facete [witty] epigram of Maximilianus Urentius, what's the difference? (p. 88)

However, Burton is aware of the use as well as abuse of medicine and diplomatically and good-humouredly restrains himself from further attacks on the profession with a 'counter-snarle':

But I will urge these cavilling and contumelious arguments no farther, <u>lest some physician should mistake me, and deny me physic when I am sick</u>: for my part, I am well persuaded of physic: I can distinguish the abuse from the use, in this and many other arts and sciences. (p. 89)

Keats's reading of Burton evidently unloosed memories of his own former profession, which were still present in his ongoing, lifelong pre-occupation with ways in which poetry could be a healing agent. The second 'Hyperion' fragment, *The Fall of Hyperion. A Dream*, posits a holistic and constitutional way of healing by beginning with the sickness of the mind registered upon the body and concluding that both the physician and the poet play curative roles of body and mind respectively: 'sure a poet is a sage, | A humanist, physician to all men'.[47]

Reading as a Poet

I am convinced more and more every day that (excepting the human friend the philosopher) a fine writer is the most genuine Being in the World – Shakespeare and the paradise Lost every day become greater wonders to me – I look upon fine Phrases like a Lover . . .[48]

So wrote Keats to Bailey in August 1819 from Winchester, announc-ing to Bailey that he has 'written 1500 Lines . . . two Tales, one from Boccaccio call'd the Pot of Basil; and another call'd Lamia (half fin-ished) . . .', and he mentions also both 'Hyperion' and the play *Otho the Great*. The fact that he does not mention Burton as a 'fine writer' may be because he counts him as 'human friend the philosopher', and because he writes prose, but in singling out many words and phrases in *The Anatomy* Keats is equally displaying his love for 'fine Phrases'. As Gittings describes, 'It is clear that Keats marked his copy of Burton as much for the *curiosa felicitas* of the words as for their meaning'.[49] He alights upon *bons mots*, inventive and arresting language, poeticisms and lyrical expressions, cryptic epigrams such as '<u>He that will avoid trouble must avoid the world</u> (Eusebeius . . .)' (p. 414), and poetic descriptions like '<u>the very blood-hound of beauty</u>' (p. 345).

It hardly matters, for example, what is meant by Burton's 'great Zanzummins, or gigantical Anakims, heavy, vast, barbarous lubbers' (p. 11), or '*some scavenger or prick-louse tailors*' (p. 279), for the words alone are enough to catch the poet's attention. The onomatopoeia caught his eye and he underlined, 'let drums beat on, trumpets sound taratantara' (p. 74). 'The hickhop' (p. 365) is Burton's distinctive spelling of 'hiccup'. Keats side-marks passages of sustained denunciation and invective: '*no sharkers, no cony-catchers, no prowlers, no smell-feasts, praters, panders, parasites, bawds, drunkards, whoremasters; necessity and defect compel them to be honest*' (84). Of dancing Burton writes kinaesthetically, '*and it was a pleasant sight to see those pretty knots, and swimming figures*' (p. 277). Burton is full of colourful invective such as 'nought but his *imperfections are in our eyes, he is a base knave, a devil, a monster, a caterpillar, a viper, a hog-rubber, &c*' (p. 170). As a poet who had written a whole romantic epic on the moon Keats evidently found noteworthy Burton's rhetorical question which keeps things in a more sardonic perspective, 'Doth the moon care for the barking of a dog?' (p. 79), and similarly on love he underlines 'But to enlarge or illustrate this power and effects of love, is to set a candle in the sun' (p. 207). As one who himself tells 'a doubtful tale from faery land' ('Lamia'), we find Keats marking Burton's '*You have heard my tale: but alas it is but a tale, a mere fiction, 'twas never so, never like to be, and so let it rest*' (p. 70, double side-marked). He is struck by the rising cadence and celebration of nature when Burton expansively waxes lyrical:

> I live and breathe *under that glorious heaven, that august capitol of nature, enjoy the brightness of stars, that clear light of sun and moon, those infinite creatures, plants, birds, beasts, fishes, herbs, all that sea and land afford, far surpassing all that art and opulentia can give.* (p. 29)

And he appreciates the suspended anticipation of Burton's periodic sentence in praise of nature in all its plenitude:

> *Whiteness in the lily, red in the rose, purple in the violet, a lustre in all things without life, the clear light of the moon, the bright beams of the sun, splendour of gold, purple, sparkling diamond, the excellent feature of the horse, the majesty of the lion, the colour of birds, peacock's tails, the silver scales of fish, we behold with singular delight and admiration.* (p. 218)

By his acts of selection, Keats is constructing Burton as a witty word-player, and at least on occasions rising to the heights of a lyrical prose-poet.

Keats clearly enjoyed Burton's conversational rhetoric when in full flight, for example in using relentless repetition of the phrase 'ride on' as a narrative device in describing a character who acts like a bad Samaritan, ignoring pleas for help in his determination to 'ride on':

> *"Show some pity for Christ's sake, pity a sick man, an old man," &c., he cares not, <u>ride on</u>: pretend sickness, inevitable loss of limbs, goods, plead suretyship, or shipwreck, fires, common calamities, show thy wants and imperfections,.. thou art a counterfeit crank, a cheater, he is not touched with it, pauper . . . <u>ride on</u>, he takes no notice of it. Put up a supplication to him in the name of a thousand orphans, a hospital, a spittle, a prison, as he goes by, they cry out to him for aid, <u>ride on</u> . . . he cares not, let them eat stones, devour themselves with vermin, rot in their own dung, he cares not. Show him a decayed haven, a bridge, a school, a fortification, etc., or some public work, <u>ride on; good your worship, your honour, for God's sake, your country's sake, ride on</u>.* (p. 186)

As satirist there are frequent touches in Burton which anticipate Swift's trenchant view of bodily imperfection, for example in the latter's hideous description in *Gulliver's Travels* of 'Struldbrugs' who, achieving immortality as they desire, cannot escape continual and inevitable human aging and physical decay. In Burton's eyes, 'decrepit' males lusting after young women are just as pathetically deluded:

> <u>How many decrepit, hoary, harsh, writhen, bursten-bellied, crooked, toothless, bald, blear-eyed, impotent, rotten, old men shall you see flickering still in every place? One gets him a young wife, another a courtesan, and when he can scarce lift his leg over a sill, and hath one foot already in Charon's boat,</u> *when he hath the trembling in his joints, the gout in his feet, a perpetual rheum in his head, "a continuate cough," his sight fails him, thick of hearing, his breath stinks, all his moisture is dried up and gone, may not spit from him, a very child again, that cannot dress himself, or cut his own meat, yet he will be dreaming of, and honing after wenches, what can be more unseemly?* (p. 207)

It is the linguistic fertility as much as the mordant content which runs through such passages and attracts Keats's attention:

> <u>A filthy knave, a deformed quean, a crooked carcass, a mawkin, a witch, a rotten post, a hedgestake may be so set out and tricked up, that it shall</u> *make as fair a show, as much enamour as the rest: many a silly fellow is so taken.* (p. 247)

Although often as critical of women's physicality as men's, small details can bring alive Burton's more complimentary descriptions of them, with phrases evidently appreciated by Keats: '*A little soft hand, pretty little mouth, small, fine, long fingers*' (p. 234); 'yellow-haired, of <u>a wheat colour,</u> but of a most amiable and piercing eye' (p. 239); '*with a regaining retreat, a gentle reluctancy, a smiling threat, a pretty pleasant peevishness*' (p. 271). Along the same lines but more comprehensively, we find this description, Keats side-marking and carefully underlining the woman's English 'hands':

> But be she fair indeed, golden-haired, as Anacreon his Bathillus, (to examine particulars) she have ... *a pure sanguine complexion, little mouth, coral lips, white teeth, soft and plump neck, body, hands, feet, all fair and lovely to behold, composed of all graces, elegances, an absolute piece, Let her head be from Prague, paps out of Austria, belly from France, back from Brabant, <u>hands</u> out of England, feet from Rhine, buttocks from Switzerland, let her have the Spanish gait, the Venetian tire, Italian compliment and endowments* ... (p. 374)

But criticism is more typical of Burton's jaundiced eye, and it is the passing of time which is regarded as the ever-present threat to young beauty, a perception regarded by both Burton and Keats as a major element in a melancholy outlook:

> child-bearing, old age, that tyrant time will turn Venus to Erinnys; raging time, care, rivels her upon a sudden; after she hath been married a small while, and the black ox hath trodden on her toe, she will be so much altered, and wax out of favour, thou wilt not know her. <u>*One grows too fat, another too lean, &c., modest Matilda, pretty pleasing Peg, sweet-singing Susan, mincing merry Moll, dainty dancing Doll, neat Nancy, jolly Joan, nimble Nell, kissing Kate, bouncing Bess, with black eyes, fair Phyllis, with fine white hands, fiddling Frank, tall Tib, slender Sib, &c.,*</u> *will quickly lose their grace, grow fulsome, stale, sad, heavy, dull, sour, and all at last out of fashion* ... *Those fair sparkling eyes will look dull, her soft coral lips will be pale, dry, cold, rough, and blue, her skin rugged, that soft and tender superficies will be hard and harsh, her whole complexion change in a moment, and as Matilda writ to King John.*
>
> > *I am not now as when thou saw'st me last,*
> > *That favour soon is vanished and past;*
> > <u>*That rosie blush lapt in a lily vale,*</u>
> > <u>*Now is with morphew overgrown and pale.*</u>

By turns bemused and dismayed by the materiality of the body, Burton and Keats seem to have shared the 'anatomist's' attitude that beneath the skin lies a skull, and that youthful beauty cannot last. I quote at length, as the sections on the whole page are sporadically side-lined and underlined by Keats:

> To conclude with Chrysostom, 'When thou seest a fair and beautiful person, a brave Bonaroba, a bella donna ... a comely woman, having bright eyes, a merry countenance, a shining lustre in her look, a pleasant grace, <u>wringing thy soule</u>, and increasing thy concupiscence; bethink with

thyself that it is but earth thou lovest, a mere excrement, which so vexeth thee, which thou so admirest, and thy raging soul will be at rest. Take her skin from her face, and thou shalt see all loathsomeness under it, that beauty is a superficial skin and bones, nerves, sinews: suppose her sick, now rivelled, hoary-headed, hollow-cheeked, old; within she is full of filthy phlegm, stinking, putrid, excremental stuff: snot and snivel in her nostrils, spittle in her mouth, water in her eyes, what filth in her brains' &c. Or take her at best, and look narrowly upon her in the light, stand near her, nearer yet, thou shalt perceive almost as much, and love less . . . [The] spectator shall find many faults in physiognomy, and ill colour: if form, one side of the face likely bigger than the other, or crooked nose, bad eyes, prominent veins, concavities about the eyes, wrinkles, pimples, red streaks, freckles, hairs, warts, neves, inequalities, roughness, scabredity, paleness, yellow-ness, <u>and as many colours as are in a turkicock's neck</u>, many indecorums in their other parts . . . one leers, another frowns, a third gapes, squints, &c.' And 'tis true that he saith . . . seldom shall you find an absolute face without fault, as I have often observed; not in the face alone is this defect or disproportion to be found; but in all the other parts, of body and mind; she is fair, indeed, but foolish; pretty, comely, and decent, of a majestical pres-ence, but peradventure, imperious, dishonest, *acerba, iniqua*, self-willed: *she is rich, but deformed; hath a sweet face, but bad carriage, no bringing up, a rude and wanton flirt; a neat body she hath, but it is a nasty quean otherwise, a very slut, of a bad kind. As flowers in a garden have colour some, but no smell, others have a fragrant smell, but are unseemly to the eye;* one is unsavoury to the taste as rue, as bitter as wormwood, and yet a most medicinal cordial flower, most acceptable to the stomach; so are men and women; one is well qualified, but of ill proportion, poor and base: a good eye she hath, but a bad hand and foot . . . a fine leg, bad teeth, a vast body, &c. Examine all parts of body and mind, I advise thee to inquire of all. *See her angry, merry, laugh, weep, hot, cold, sick, sullen, dressed, undressed, in all attires, sites, gestures, passions, eat her meals, &c., and in some of these you will surely dislike.* (pp. 375–7)

Not surprisingly, such rejective perceptions are a disincentive to mar-riage, in Burton's rather cloistered worldview:

> *If women in general be so bad (and men worse than they) what a hazard is it to marry? where shall a man find a good wife, or a woman a good husband? . . . The worldly cares, miseries, discontents, that accompany marriage, I pray you learn of them that have experience, for I have none.* (p. 380)

Unfortunately, just as common in Burton's time (and to some extent in Keats's) is Hamlet's brand of invective in imputing duplicity to women, but less common is Burton's colourful imagery to make his points, which is noticed by Keats. Quoting Aristaenetus, he writes,

> [Women] wipe away their tears like sweat, <u>weep with one eye, laugh with the other</u>; or as children weep and cry, they can both together.

Care not for women's tears, I counsel thee,
They teach their eyes as much to weep as see.
<u>And as much pity is to be taken of a woman weeping, as of a goose going
barefoot</u>. (p. 283)

Reading as a poet, Keats is on the lookout for any comments on the
subject of poets and poetry themselves: 'Death himself, when he should
have stroken a sweet young virgin with his dart, he fell in love with the
object. Many more such could I relate <u>which are to be believed with a
poetical faith</u>' (p. 225) (also underlined by George Taylor in his edition);
*'The poets therefore did well to feign all shepherds lovers, to give them-
selves to songs and dalliances, because they lived such idle lives'* (p. 214).
Keats places a cross beside this passage by Burton: 'I say nothing all this
while of idols themselves that have committed idolatry in this kind, of
looking-glasses, that have been rapt in love (if you will believe poets)'
(p. 224), and comments sarcastically at the bottom of the page on how
Burton himself is guilty of such 'idolatry': 'How is he caught by his own
birdlime!' (possibly recalling *Much Ado About Nothing*, 'She's lim'd, I
warrant you! We have caught her . . .' [3.1.104]). Burton himself can be
ironic and perhaps self-deprecating about poets:

> So Siracides himself speaks as much as may be for and against women, so
> doth almost every philosopher plead pro and con, every poet thus argues the
> case (<u>though what cares *vulgus nominum* what they say?</u>) (p. 417)

There are innumerable other references to 'feigning' poets and quotations from poetry which are not marked by Keats, but the ones that are,
indicate a major interest of Burton, poetry's links with melancholy, as
do the items listed in his index to the *Anatomy* ('The Table'), 'Poets why
poor | Poetry a symptom of lovers | Poetical cures of love-melancholy'
(p. 609). Love as inspiration for poets gets Burton's full treatment,
making even rustics eloquent:

> *Petrarch's Laura made him so famous, Astrophel's Stella, and Jovianus
> Pontanus' mistress was the cause of his roses, violets, lilies . . . and the rest of
> his poems; why are Italians at this day generally so good poets and painters?
> Because every man of any fashion amongst them hath his mistress. The very
> rustics and <u>hog-rubbers,</u> Menalcas and Corydon, qui faetant de stercore
> equino [who reek of horse dung], those fulsome knaves, if once they taste of
> this love-liquor, are inspired in an instant. Instead of those accurate emblems,
> curious impresses, gaudy masques, tilts, tournaments, &c., they have their
> wakes, Whitsun ales, shepherd's feasts, meetings on holidays, country dances,
> roundelays, writing their names on trees, true lover's knots, pretty gifts . . .*
> Instead of odes, epigrams and elegies, &c., they have their ballads, country
> tunes, <u>*O the broom, the bonny, bonny broom*</u>, ditties and songs, <u>*Bess a belle,
> she doth excel*</u>, – they must write likewise and indite all in rhyme . . . But I

conclude there is no end of love's symptoms, 'tis a bottomless pit. (pp. 343–6 *passim*)

Like George Taylor but not so frequently, Keats spotted quotations which either had literary sources or were repeated by later writers. Some of his annotations are of this kind: Ben Jonson (p. 297), *Romeo and Juliet* (p. 264), Massinger (pp. 404 and 444), the Bible (pp. 513 and 536), Malthus (p. 409), Isaac Bickerstaff (p. 281), and Sterne (pp. 14 and 99). On p. 225 he side-marks and places a cross in the margin against '*for he thought it impossible for any man living to see her and contain himself.* The very fame of beauty will fetch them to it many miles off (such an attractive power this loadstone hath)'. Keats adds a comment at the bottom of the page 'Witness Mary of Buttermere, Knighton Sally'. The first of these was Mary Robinson (1778–1837) who gained fame as 'the Maid of Buttermere'. She was known to Coleridge and mentioned in Wordsworth's *The Prelude* as a paragon of 'unspoiled' rustic virtue, originally a shepherdess but so beautiful that she was known far and wide and became a social celebrity. The Fish Inn in Buttermere, Cumbria, run by her family, became the destination of secular pilgrims just to glimpse her. After marrying an imposter and forger she finally 'won the sympathy and admiration of poets, dramatists, journalists, and biographers' on her death.[50] Presumably there was another with the same loadstone-like 'fame of beauty', called Sally who lived in Knighton (a small town on the Welsh border, later given celebrity by Houseman's 'The Carpenter's Son' in *A Shropshire Lad*), but I cannot track her down.

Melancholy and Love

It is emerging that the subject of Keats reading Burton is a perfect example for reader-response theory in several ways. He clearly reads with an openness that suggests his own ideal of 'Negative Capability', through his markings steadily constructing Burton's own, many-sided literary personality and tones which are by turns witty, wry, mischievous, stylistically masterful and linguistically sprightly, earthy, satirical, sceptical, angry, scholarly, poetical, forensic. The impression of Burton's weighty tunnel vision and his overload of authorities and Latin quotations is qualified by drawing attention to the playfulness. Melancholy cannot be such a debilitating disease if it can produce the playful prose and story-telling that Keats finds in the *Anatomy*.

At the same time, this all-inclusive accumulation of detail is also

Keats's own active self-fashioning as a poet, reading as a poet and drawing from the text what is professionally of interest to him. We detect a creative continuum between the functions of the reader and the poet when the two elide: some passages selected by Keats seem to be ones that feed into his own poetry, either directly or indirectly. It is hard not to recognise a touch of Porphryo's stealthy approach in 'St Agnes Eve' in Burton's words:

> *is not somebody in that great chest, or behind the door, or hangings, or in some of those barrels? may not a man steal in at the window with a ladder of ropes, or come down the chimney, have a false key, or get in when he is asleep? If a mouse do but stir, or the wind blow, a casement clatter, that's the villain, there he is.* (p. 448)

Under the section headed 'Symptoms or signs of Love Melancholy, in Body, Mind, good, bad &c.' Burton tabulates first the female symptoms anticipating Keats's Isabella: 'they pine away, and look ill with waking, cares, sighs . . . With groans, griefs, sadness, dullness . . . want of appetite, &c.' (p. 290) which Burton explains by referring to a medical authority as caused by

> the distraction of the spirits the liver doth not perform his part, nor turns the aliment into blood as it ought, and for that cause the members are weak for want of sustenance, they are lean and pine, as the herbs of my garden do this month of May, for want of rain. The green sickness therefore often happeneth to young women . . . (p. 291)

Keats does not mark this, but he certainly read it, as he shows by side-lining a poem on the following page, detailing male symptoms of love melancholy:

> *His sleep, his meat, his drink, in him bereft,*
> *That lean he waxeth, and dry as a shaft,*
> *His eyes hollow and grisly to behold,*
> *His hew pale and ashen to unfold,*
> *And solitary he was ever alone,*
> *And waking all the night making moan.* (p. 293)

We seem here to be beside that lake in 'La Belle Dame sans Merci. A Ballad', observing the knight-at-arms, 'Alone and palely loitering' and 'so haggard and so woe-begone', though it is the man in Burton who is 'all the night making moan' rather than Keats's Spenserian 'faery' belle dame who 'made sweet moan'. Keats originally wrote 'starved lips' of the knight, following Burton's *'His sleep, his meat, his drink, in him bereft'*. Sinson comes close to being categorical in concluding that '"La Belle Dame" is almost certainly derived directly from Burton',[51] pointing out that there are also passages that 'echo Burton too closely to be coincidences' in the journal-letter to the George Keatses on 21 April 1819 in which the poem is transcribed, alongside several others including 'Ode to Psyche', and in which he explains the 'vale of Soul-making'. Sinson also points to another section of Burton, this time in Book 1, which adds weight to the notion that Keats had read this volume too. The passage (referring to Homer's *The Iliad*) describes symptoms not so much of love-melancholy but melancholy in general in its 'cold' and watery form:

> That wandered in the woods, sad all alone Forsaking men's society, making great moan; they delight in floods and waters, desert places, to walk alone in orchards, gardens, private walks, back lanes; averse from company, or confluence of waters, all day long and all day night . . . They are much given to weeping and delight in waters, ponds, pools . . . they are pale of colour, slothful, apt to sleep, much troubled with the headache.[52]

There are several literary allusions in the densely packed 'La Belle Dame', and Keats himself mentions to Fanny Brawne 'an oriental tale of a very beautiful colour', in which 'a city of melancholy men' had been made so by 'a most enchanting Lady' who orders them to shut their eyes, and on awakening 'The remembrance of this Lady and their delights lost beyond all recovery render them melancholy ever after'.[53] Another likely source seems especially suggestive as a companion to Burton's, namely Spenser's depiction of Prince Arthur's vision or dream of spending the night with the 'Queene of Faeries'. Burton himself quotes from *The Faerie Queene*, and lists Spenser as among many prototypical 'modern poets' of his day who deal with love-melancholy (p. 342). Here is Spenser's passage in full:

> For-wearied with my sports, I did alight
> From loftie steed, and downe to sleepe me layd;
> The verdant gras my couch did goodly dight,
> And pillow was my helmet faire displayd:
> Whiles euery sence the humour sweet embayd,
> And slombring soft my hart did steale away,
> Me seemed, by my side a royall Mayd
> Her daintie limbes full softly down did lay:
> So faire a creature yet saw neuer sunny day.
>
> Most goodly glee and louely blandishment
> She to me made, and bad me loue her deare,
> For dearely sure her loue was to me bent,
> As when iust time expired should appeare.
> But whether dreames delude, or true it were,
> Was neuer hart so rauisht with delight,
> Ne liuing man like words did euer heare,

As she to me deliuered all that night;
And at her parting said, She Queene of Faeries hight.

When I awoke, and found her place deuoyd,
And nought but pressed gras, where she had lyen,
I sorrowed all so much, as earst I ioyd,
And washed all her place with watry eyen.
From that day forth I lou'd that face diuine;
From that day forth I cast in carefull mind,
To seeke her out with labour, and long tyne,
And neuer vow to rest, till her I find,
Nine monethes I seeke in vaine yet ni'll that vow vnbind.

Thus as he spake, his visage wexed pale,
And chaunge of hew great passion did bewray;
Yet still he stroue to cloke his inward bale,
And hide the smoke, that did his fire display [54]

The context of this passage in *The Faerie Queene* gives a more positive gloss than Burton's, since the predicted marriage between Arthur and Gloriana is regarded by Spenser as ideal, while Burton's males in love are ridiculed. The coexistence of both sources behind Keats's poem can only add to its mystery.

There is another, amusing piece of evidence, not elsewhere noticed to my knowledge, that Keats had Burton's *Anatomy* in mind, however unconsciously, when writing in 'La Belle Dame', 'And there I shut her wild wild eyes with kisses four'. After transcribing the poem for his brother and sister-in-law, he writes facetiously:

Why four kisses – you will say – why four because I wish to restrain the headlong impetuosity of my Muse – she would have fain said 'score' without hurting the rhyme – but we must temper the Imagination as the Critics say with Judgment. I was obliged to choose an even number that both eyes might have fair play; and to speak truly I think two a piece quite sufficient – Suppose I had said seven; there would have been three and a half a piece – a very awkward affair – and well got out of on my side – (*JKL* 2, 97)

While undoubtedly typical of Keats's own sense of humour, it may have had its inspiration from the following, equally fanciful sequence from Burton (I silently delete the many Latin quotations and references, to abbreviate this lengthy passage and to foreground its content):

"They breathe out their souls and spirits together with their kisses," saith Balthazar Castilio, "change hearts and spirits, and mingle affections as they do kisses, and it is rather a connection of the mind than of the body." And although these kisses be delightsome and pleasant, Ambrosial kisses, sweeter than nectar, balsam, honey, love-dropping kisses; for

> *The gilliflower, the rose is not so sweet,*
> *As sugared kisses be when lovers meet;*

Yet they leave an irksome impression, like that of aloes or gall,

> At first Ambrose itself was not sweeter,
> At last black hellebore was not so bitter.
> They are deceitful kisses,
> Why dost within thine arms me lap,
> And with false kisses me entrap.
>
> They are destructive, and the more the worse: There be honest kisses, I
> deny not, friendly kisses, modest kisses, vestal-virgin kisses, officious and
> ceremonial kisses, &c., kissing and embracing are proper gifts of Nature to a
> man; but these are too lascivious kisses, too continuate and too violent, they
> cling like ivy, close as an oyster, bill as doves, meretricious kisses, biting of
> lips, kisses as she gave to Gyton, innumerable kisses, &c. More than kisses,
> or too homely kisses: ... with such other obscenities *that vain lovers use,*
> *which are abominable and pernicious. If every kiss a man gives his wife after*
> *marriage*, be a mortal sin, what shall become of all such immodest kisses and
> obscene actions, the forerunners of brutish lust, if not lust itself! (pp. 266–7)

Itemising twenty kisses in one passage seems to reflect the 'headlong
impetuosity' of Burton's 'muse', perhaps evidence of the celibate,
monkish academic indulging in wish-fulfilment, and impishly camou-
flaging his own lascivious 'lust' beneath a barrage of learned Latinisms
and scholarly authorities. Keats seems in his markings to be in joking
dialogue with Burton.

'La Belle Dame' inevitably raises the vexed question of Keats's divided
attitude to women in general, which is an issue in Burton as well. Since
the rise of feminist criticism in the 1980s, it has become a commonplace
that he regularly expressed a relatively traditional masculinist view of
women as polarised between ethereal angel and demonic enchantress.[55]
(Ironically, at the same time contemporary critics, including Hazlitt,
condemned his own style as 'effeminate'.) The bifocal division seems to
have had both biographical and literary sources. He wrote to his sister-
in-law Georgiana of the charismatic presence of the Indian Jane Cox, 'as
an eternal Being I love the thought of you. I should like her to ruin me,
and I should like you to save me'.[56] Of the effect on him of being in the
presence of both Jane Cox and Fanny Brawne, Keats used the vocabulary of anxiety, 'dissolving' with a 'loss of self' or 'loss of identity', being
'ravished' and 'absorbed', but wishing to 'not give way to it'.[57] He was
aware of, and made uncomfortable by, these feelings:

> I am certain I have not a right feeling towards Women – at this moment I am
> striving to be just to them but I cannot – Is it because they fall so far beneath

my Boyish imagination? When I was a Schoolboy I though[t] a fair Woman a pure Goddess, my mind was a soft nest in which some of them slept though she knew it not – I have no right to expect more than their reality . . . When I am among Women I have evil thoughts, malice spleen – I cannot speak or be silent – I am full of Suspicions and therefore listen to no thing – I am in a hurry to be gone – You must be charitable and put all this perversity to my being disappointed since Boyhood . . .[58]

The final phrase would seem to refer to his mother's remarriage and defection from her children, after Keats's father died. He regarded his disillusioned discomfort as immature ('Boyish') but entrenched in his mind since childhood, seeking ways to 'cure' it:

The only way is to find the root of evil, and so cure it "with backward mutters of dissevering Power" that is so difficult a thing; for an obstinate Prejudice can seldom be produced but from a gordian complication of feelings, which must take time to unravel[ed] and care to keep unravelled.[59]

In his poems of love, his male protagonists demonstrate similarly divided emotional reactions, and the common theme of his attitude to women is a 'shifting between veneration and apprehension'.[60] In 'Lamia' and 'La Belle Dame' especially, the ambivalence is expressed as a contrast between woman as angel and woman as demon, while Isabella and Madeline ('so pure a thing, so free from mortal taint') escape the ambiguous status, but could be equally stereotyped as passive victims, insulated from reality in dreams. In terms of literary influences, Burton certainly aided and abetted the divided view of women, but in Keats's earlier reading it was Spenser's *The Faerie Queene* which provided the main precedent. His women are divided between the holiness of Una on the one hand, and the deceiving Duessa, enchantress and *femme fatale* on the other:

Her nether parts misshapen, monstruous,
Were hidd in water, that I could not see,
But they did seeme more foule and hideous,
Then womans shape man would believe to bee.

                                                    (1.2.41–4)

Even if Lamia is not a mortal woman, and the implied seductress in 'La Belle Dame Sans Merci' is not hiding 'parts misshapen', yet the two poems in their different ways betray aspects of the congenital wariness of women shared by both Burton and Keats.

As Gittings, Sinson and Barnard all point out, it is surprising that Keats did not publish 'La Belle Dame' in *1820*, especially since there is a kind of internal cross reference when Porphyro in 'The Eve of St Agnes' plays on the lute 'an ancient ditty, long since mute, | In Provence call'd,

"La belle dame sans mercy"', referring this time to the medieval French poem by Alain Chartier. Its inclusion would certainly have neatly fitted the theme of melancholy which I am pursuing here, and also the book's timeline, since the poem had been written in April 1819 at the same time as the 'great' odes. It was published in *The Indicator* on 10 May 1820, under the *nom de plume* 'Caviare', possibly ironising and distancing the work as though Keats did not wish to claim public authorship of a poem which he may have thought as 'smokable' as 'Isabella'. It was republished posthumously in 1848, and revisions between three different versions, not all improvements, may indicate that he was never quite satisfied with it. Maybe its fragmentary air of secrecy, subjective experience, and unexplained enigma – the very qualities in the poem which appeal to modern readers – struck him as too indeterminate for a 'ballad' where clearer narrative closure might be expected.

Nonetheless, the exclusion of 'La Belle Dame' still seems puzzling, especially since the brief and (one would think) inferior work written at the same time and appearing in the same letter to his brother George, 'Song of Four Faeries', seems inexplicably to have made it as far as the final cut for inclusion in the 1820 volume. According to a note made by Woodhouse on his transcript, it was 'Corrected, by Keats's copy for the press'.[61] The subtitle, 'Fire, Air, Earth, and Water', connects it with the taxonomy of the humours which Burton presupposes in *The Anatomy of Melancholy*. The element of fire was associated with yellow bile, air with blood, earth with black bile and water with phlegm. These humoural equations do seem to be in play in Keats's poem, since Salamander hails 'Happy, happy glowing fire', Zephyr 'Fragrant air!', Dusketha (melancholy) begins 'Let me to my glooms retire!', and Breama, 'I to green-weed rivers bright'. The short work is in the form of a rather inconclusive debate between the four 'characters'. Gittings notes that both 'La Belle Dame' and the 'Song' seem to be inspired by the same passages in Burton's *Anatomy* quoted above (pp. 280–4), and continues: 'Here, of course, is the idea of the *Song of Four Faeries*; but more particularly Burton deals in these pages, which Keats was reading, with those who suffer from the symptoms of the cold "humour" of melancholy'.[62] The debate between the fairies is concluded with the development of an affinity between Salamander and Dusketha, implying allegorically an ideal love couple, while the fairies representing air and water go their separate ways. The description of Dusketha as 'adder-eyed' and 'Freckle-winged and lizard-sided!' suggests a link with Lamia, while the airy and watery characters seem types of the lovers in 'La Belle Dame', melancholy but inactive. Based on this connection, the serious consideration Keats gave to including 'Song of Four Faeries' lends supporting evidence to the argument here being advanced that melancholy and Burton are central reference points running through the 1820 volume. However, the thematic reasons for inclusion seem to have been outweighed by the poem's qualitative slightness, a decision which few would regret.

The proximity of love to degrading lust seems intellectually to dismay Keats in a personal way, as we find in one of his most notorious annotations. In Burton's frequent rants about lasciviousness Keats glimpses at least a cultural contradiction in notions of love, sexual and religious. His extended annotation on pages 166–7 comes alongside Burton's relatively orthodox summary of Plato's explanation of love as engendered in the perception of beauty which leads to virtue, but Keats seems to be thinking more about the division than about Burton's description itself:

> Here is the old plague spot; the pestilence, the raw scrofula. I mean that there is nothing disgraces me in my own eyes so much as being one of a race of eyes nose and mouth beings in a planet call'd the earth who all from Plato to Wesley have always mingled goatish winnyish lustful love with the abstract adoration of the deity. I don't understand Greek – is the love of God and the Love of women express'd by the same word in Greek? I hope my little mind is wrong – if not I could – Has Plato separated these loves? Ha! I see how they endeavor to divide – but there appears to be a horrid relationship.

The outburst reflects some sexual revulsion in his own attitudes, but more intriguingly it appears beside Burton's semi-scholarly meditation on Plato's theory of love, the paradox that *agape* and *eros* stem from the same impulse: 'Plato calls it the great devil, for its vehemency, and sovereignty over all other passions, and defines it an appetite, "by which we desire some good to be present"' (p. 159). The underlying philosophical point has some relevance to the depiction of love's ambiguities in 'Lamia' and possibly 'The Eve of St Agnes'. As for the vehement and apparently bitter tone of Keats's annotation, John Whale describes it as follows:

> there is a metaphysically defined disappointment: the promise of the perfectibility of the soul taken away by the animalistic tendencies of the body. The combination of soul and body is polarized as a disturbing opposition between 'lustful love' and 'abstract adoration'. Keats articulates a profound sense of personal abjection – 'disgraces me in my own eyes' – with a universalizing sense of shame which takes us beyond misogyny into a realm of Swiftian misanthropy.[63]

But then again, if read in context, Keats's comment need not be so bitter and personal as this suggests, but more of a meditation on the apparent moral contradictions in Plato's theory of love, as Rachel Schulkins tends to suggest when considering the intriguing annotation:

> Keats rejects the artificiality and the embellished ceremonial gestures claimed in the name of romance. He sees men as the victims of their own romantic, infantile behaviour, while women are the mere passive objects of false adoration.[64]

As with most subjects involving Keats, we must accept a degree of ambiguity in his annotation, and it remains an open question whether he is writing as a suffering lover, as an observant poet, or as a philologist pondering platonic theory and the Greek language. Coincidentally, the period during which he was reading Burton also coincided with the time of most volatile and intense relationship with Fanny Brawne. Although Keats may be commenting directly on Plato's theory, the spirit of striking distaste evidenced in 'the old scrofula' note also intersects with the more negative side of both Burton's and Keats's view of relations between men and women, and ambiguity about women in general.

In Burton's eyes, love melancholy is diverse in symptoms and dangerous in consequences. Using as examples the Trojan wars and the fates of Antony and Cleopatra, Burton warns of dangers for the nation of the kind of love that 'furiously rages' in public figures, likened to 'madness, to make away with themselves and others, violent death; the prognostication is, they will either run mad, or die. *For if this passion continue,'* saith Aelian Montaltus, *'it makes the blood hot, thick, and black; and if the inflammation get into the brain, with continual meditation and waking, it so dries it up, that madness follows, or else they make away themselves'* (p. 347). He therefore proposes different cures for different types of love. Keats paid attention to Burton's section on *'Cure of Love-Melancholy, by Labour, Diet, Physic, Fasting, &c.'* He side-marks the section proclaiming that *'Fasting is an all-sufficient remedy of itself'* (p. 352) and notes Burton's quotation concerning extreme bodily deprivation in some societies, such as that of 'Indian Brahmins':

> *If imprisonment and hunger will not take them down, according to the directions of that Theban Crates, 'time must wear it out; if time will not, the last refuge is a halter.'* <u>But this, you will say, is comically spoken</u>. (p. 353)

To cure lust, Burton advises, 'all lascivious meats must be forsaken. *Those opposite meats which ought to be used are cucumbers, melons, purslane, water-lilies, rue, woodbine, ammi, lettuce, which Lemnius so much commends'* (p. 354). Keats side-marks with what looks like an exclamation mark, the sentence in which Burton prescribes his favoured remedy for any form of melancholy, hellebore: '*Amatus Lusitanus cured a young Jew, that was almost mad for love, with the syrup of hellebore, and such other evacuations and purges which are usually prescribed to black choler*' (p. 355). Other emotional problems attending the lover can be antidoted in more behavioural ways, by employing pleasurable distractions (quoting Vives):

> A lover that hath as it were lost himself through impotency, impatience, must be called home as a traveller, by music, feasting, good wine, if need be to drunkenness itself, which many so much commend for the easing of the mind, all kinds of sports and merriments, to see fair pictures, hangings, buildings, *pleasant fields, orchards, gardens, groves, ponds, pools, rivers, fishing, fowling, hawking, hunting, to hear merry tales, and pleasant discourse, reading, to use exercise till he sweat, that new spirits may succeed, or by some vehement affection or contrary passion to be diverted till he be fully weaned from anger, suspicion, cares, fears,* &c., ... *And as the melody of music, merriment, singing, dancing, doth augment the passion of some lovers, as Avicenna notes, so it expelleth it in others, and doth very much good. These things must be warily applied, as the parties' symptoms vary, and as they shall stand variously affected.* (pp. 354–5)

Among remedies for love, Burton also includes a short section on 'Philters, Magical and Poetical Cures' (Subsect. IV), but Keats no doubt enjoyed reading as much as Burton writing, the next Subsection, '*The last and best Cure of Love-Melancholy, is to let them have their Desire*'. 'The last refuge and surest remedy, to be put in practice in the *utmost place, when no other means will take effect, is to let them go together, and enjoy one another*' (p. 392). Keats places what again looks like an exclamation mark beside 'Areteus, an old author ... hath an instance of a young man, when no other means could prevail, was so speedily relieved ...', and continues underlining, '"they may then kiss and coll, lye and look babies in one anothers eyes," as their sires before them did, they may then satiate themselves with love's pleasures, which they have so long wished and expected' (pp. 392–3). It is the 'solution sweet' provided by the poet in 'The Eve of St Agnes', for the ardent, lascivious Porphyro and 'perplexed' Madeline.

Keats's 'Index'

A puzzle lies at the end of Keats's copy of Burton's book. On the blank page at the end of his copy of the *Anatomy*, Keats wrote an apparent index or list for himself, pointing to pages that for some reason interest him in the volume. Most deal with love stories and some with tyrants, but their general, let alone specific, significance to him, and reasons why he itemises them, remain uncertain. Given that some of his notes sound like titles for stories, and that the 'Lamia' page is among them, it is tempting to see them as narratives which Keats may have considered possible subjects for poems or even plays. I apologise for not being able to offer explanations, apart from a few speculations, but record and quote at some length from them, in case others may offer enlightenment. There is a limit to how much we can glean from looking over Keats's shoulder as he reads. Admittedly, these annotations remain enigmatic, though they do at least demonstrate again how carefully Keats attended to detail in his reading.

Some in the index may give him a quick way of relocating some striking passages, as seems likely in the first, cryptically described as 'Page 200 Ione-Fredegunde-Brunhault'. Here Burton mentions some of the notoriously lustful historical figures such as the sinful citizens of Sodom and Gomorrah, Helen of Troy, 'Joanna of Naples in Italy, Fredegunde and Brunhalt in France'. These lead Burton into one of his frequent vituperations against 'burning lust, a disease, frenzy, madness, hell':

> It subverts kingdoms, overthrows cities, towns, families, mars, corrupts, and makes a massacre of men; thunder and lightning, wars, fires, plagues, have not done that mischief to mankind, as this burning lust, this brutish passion . . . Besides those daily monomachies, murders, effusion of blood, rapes, riot, and immoderate expense, to satisfy their lusts, beggary, shame, loss, torture, punishment, disgrace, loathsome diseases that proceed from thence, worse than calentures and pestilent fevers, those often gouts, pox, arthritis, palsies, cramps, sciatica, convulsions, aches, combustions, &c., which torment the body, <u>that feral melancholy which crucifies the soul in this life</u>, and everlastingly torments in the world to come. (p. 200)

Quite a few of Keats's markings and annotations come at such points where Burton lets fly at lust, '<u>that feral melancholy</u>', and it may be either the forceful language or the jaundiced attitudes towards 'that raw scrofula', that drew Keats's attention.

The second item in Keats's index, '205 Aretine's Lucretia', dwells once again on Burton's view of insatiable lust even within marriage, this time with a misogynistic stress: he speaks of 'a wandering, extravagant, a domineering, a boundless, an irrefragable, a destructive passion' which can afflict even wives:

> Some furiously rage before they come to discretion, or age. Quartilla in Petronius never remembered she was a maid; and the wife of Bath, in Chaucer, cracks,
> Since I was twelve years old, believe,
> Husbands at Kirk-door had I five.

Aratine Lucretia sold her maidenhead a thousand times before she was twenty-four years old . . . Rahab, that harlot, began to be a professed quean at ten years of age, and was but fifteen when she hid the spies . . .

What seems to interest Burton in these examples, and perhaps also attracted Keats's attention, is the variety of manifestations of 'heroical' melancholy in love. Keats's next index entry, '217 Balthasar Castilio' deals with examples of those who fall in love without sight of the other:

Such persons commonly feign a kind of beauty to themselves; and so did those three gentlewomen in Balthazar Castilio fall in love with a young man whom they never knew, but only heard him commended: or by reading of a letter; for there is a grace cometh from hearing, as a moral philosopher informeth us, 'as well from sight; and the species of love are received into the fantasy by relation alone . . .'

However, Burton adds the conventional platonic explanation for love: *'the most familiar and usual cause of love is that which comes by sight* . . . as two sluices let in the influences of that divine, powerful, soul-ravishing, and captivating beauty'. At the least we can say that all the entries made so far by Keats relate to stories of problematical sexual matters and love's complexities.

Keats records his next entry as '228 The magic ring' and it may hold interest for more narrative reasons, perhaps as offering potential poetic treatment. Buxton Forman points out that the page number is incorrect. He does not suggest an alternative, but the reference is likely to be to Burton's pages 197–8 which deal with 'fables' of sexual relations with devils, succubi, incubi and witches, all 'mere fantasies . . . lies and tales'. These include the story of Lamia on the preceding page which Keats took as his source (also indexed). The tale of the ring is recounted by Burton at some length:

One more I will relate out of Florilegus, *ad annum* 1058, an honest historian of our nation, because he telleth it so confidently, as a thing in those days talked of all over Europe: a young gentleman of Rome, the same day that he was married, after dinner with the bride and his friends went a walking into the fields, and towards evening to the tennis-court to recreate himself; whilst he played, he put his ring upon the finger of *Venus statua* [the statue of Venus], which was thereby made in brass; after he had sufficiently played, and now made an end of his sport, he came to fetch his ring, but Venus had bowed her finger in, and he could not get it off. Whereupon loath to make his company tarry at present, there left it, intending to fetch it the next day, or at some more convenient time, went thence to supper, and so to bed. In the night, when he should come to perform those nuptial rites, Venus steps between him and his wife (unseen or felt of her), and told her that she was his wife, that he had betrothed himself unto her by that ring, which he put upon her finger: she troubled him for some following nights. He not knowing how to help himself, made his moan to one Palumbus, a learned magician in those days, who gave him a letter, and bid him at such a time of the night, in such a cross-way, at the town's end, where old Saturn would pass by with his associates in procession, as commonly he did, deliver that script with his own hands to Saturn himself; the young man of a bold spirit, accordingly did it; and when the old fiend had read it, he called Venus to him, who rode before him, and commanded her to deliver his ring, which forthwith she did, and so the gentleman was freed. (pp. 197–8)

The tale is based on the divide between the gods and mortals, as are *Endymion* and 'Lamia', and the narrative is neat enough to fuel a Keatsian sequel to these poems. He may also have had in mind the two fragments based on the Hyperion myth, given the intercession of Saturn. On the text, Keats placed crosses beside the phrases 'where old Saturn would pass by' and '[Many of those spiritual] bodies, overcome by the love of maids, and lust, failed, of whom those were born we call giants' (p. 197). Alternatively, in his index Keats may not have got the page number incorrect but the actual reference, since on his nominated page (p. 228) he underlines phrases in the literary description of doomed love (which also caught the eye of George Taylor, who side-lines them), which do not involve a 'magic ring' but list some lovers who died for love:

> Great Alexander married Roxanne, a poor man's child, only for her person. 'Twas well done of Alexander, and heroically done; I admire him for it. Orlando was mad for Angelica, and who doth not condole his mishap? Thisbe died for Pyramus, Dido for Aeneas; who doth not weep, as (before his conversion) Austin did in commiseration of her estate! she died for him; 'methinks' (as he said) *I could die for her.*

Next in Keats's list comes '330 The Sultan of Sana's wife – Lodov. Vertomannus', another tale of thwarted, obsessive love, this time based on miscegenation. Although petering out into no particular closure in Burton's telling, it is sensational enough to suggest a potential subject for a poem:

> The sultan of Sana's wife in Arabia, when she had seen Vertomannus, that comely traveller, lamented to herself in this manner, 'O God, thou hast made this man whiter than the sun, but me, mine husband, and all my children black; I would to God he were my husband, or that I had such a son;' she fell a weeping, and so impatient for love at last, . . . [she] loaded him with all the rhetoric she could,– 'grant this last request to a wretched lover.' But when he gave not consent, she would have gone with him, and left all, to be his page, his servant, or his lackey . . . so that she might enjoy him, threatening moreover to kill herself, &c. Men will do as much and more for women, spend goods, lands, lives, fortunes; kings will leave their crowns, as King John for Matilda the nun at Dunmow.

But kings in this yet privileg'd may be,
I'll be a monk so I may live with thee.

Some of Keats's indexed references are so minimally developed by Burton that the reader may be signalling his intention of following up to find out more about stories which intrigue him. The page noted by Keats as '350 Nereus' wife Chalcocondilas de reb. Turcic. P.' also deals with thwarted love. Burton quotes from Shakespeare enough times to suggest he has access to printed copies of the plays, and here he begins his list of examples by this time quoting directly: 'Whoever heard a story of more woe, | Than that of Juliet and her Romeo?'. He proceeds by telling 'love stories, all tending almost to this purpose', among them one recounting a tale involving what seems questionable morality: 'Nereus' wife, a widow, and lady of Athens, for the love of a Venetian gentleman, betrayed the city; and he for her sake murdered his wife, the daughter of a nobleman in Venice'. It is a puzzling reference, too brief to offer much by way of significance. Next, Keats's 'Chalcocondilas de reb. Turcic.' is Burton's brief footnoted reference to his source, suggesting again that Keats may have considered chasing it up to find out more. '366 Aeneas Silvius Hist. de Euryalo et Lucretia' is even more fleetingly mentioned in Burton's footnote, cited amongst examples of obsessive lovers who are 'cured' of melancholy by being married off to more accessible and compatible partners: 'After the death of Lucretia, Euryalus would admit of no comfort, till the Emperor Sigismund married him to a noble lady of his court, and so in short space he was freed'.

'404 Rodophe's shoe' is a story resembling that of Cinderella's lost 'glass slipper', concluding with a curiously irrelevant moral in Burton's account:

> *Rodophe was the fairest lady in her days in all Egypt; she went to wash her, and by chance, (her maids meanwhile looking but carelessly to her clothes) an eagle stole away one of her shoes, and laid it in Psammeticus the King of Egypt's lap at Memphis: he wondered at the excellency of the shoe and pretty foot, but more* Aquilae, factum, *at the manner of the bringing of it: and caused forthwith proclamation to be made, that she that owned that shoe should come presently to his court; the virgin came, and was forthwith married to the king. I say this was heroically done, and like a prince: I commend him for it, and all such as have means, that will either do (as he did) themselves, or so for love, &c., marry their children. If he be rich, let him take such a one as [he] wants, if she be virtuously given ...*

Here, as elsewhere, Burton's way of concluding his stories is not his strong suit since many of them end inconsequentially, as his interest in his own narration seems to wane in an eagerness to move onto the next point.

The next few entries noted by Keats deal not with love but politics and especially tyrants. It may be significant that throughout 1819 Keats was not only writing poems on love but also drama about politics, hoping *Otho the Great*, the play written in collaboration with Brown, would be accepted by a theatre, and beginning another, *King Stephen*. '425 Alex. Gaguin. Muscov. Hist. descript.' is a reference which Keats has transcribed directly from Burton's footnote to the phrase 'And what furious designs hath Jo. Basilius, that Muscovian tyrant, practised of late?'. The next reference, '463 Eumenes –', in Burton's account is a tale of violence, fraternal betrayal, and final forgiveness.

Another reference, again dealing with tyranny, is more suggestive, and may have stimulated Keats's imagination towards a new play. The indexed '575 Alphonsus King of Naples', as Buxton Forman points out, in fact occurs on page 571. This page may have caught Keats's attention partly because it has two references to Otho, and he may have been prompted to think of drama also because Burton mentions a kind of 'sequel' to *Macbeth*, quoting from one of Shakespeare's sources, Buchanan's *History of Scotland*:

> Kennetus, King of Scotland, when he had murdered his nephew Malcolm, King Duffe's son, Prince of Cumberland, and with counterfeit tears and pro-testations dissembled the matter a long time, 'at last his conscience accused him, his unquiet soul could not rest day or night, he was terrified with fearful dreams, visions, and so miserably tormented all his life.'

These characters are named here in Burton's catalogue of tyrants who came to a conscience-stricken end when they found their souls tormented for their sins: 'Tragical examples in this kind are too familiar and common: Adrian, Galba, Nero, Otho, Vitellius, Caracalla, were in such horror of conscience for their offences committed, murders, rapes, extortions, injuries, that they were weary of their lives, and could get nobody to kill them'. The reference to 'Alphonsus King of Naples' has a tick in the margin from Keats, and reads as follows:

> It is strange to read what Cominaeus hath written of Louis XI. that French King; of Charles VIII.; of Alphonsus, King of Naples; in the fury of his passion how he came into Sicily, and what pranks he played. Guicciardini, a man most unapt to believe lies, relates how that Ferdinand his father's ghost (who before had died for grief,) came and told him, that he could not resist the French King, he thought every man cried France, France; the reason of it (saith Cominaeus) was because he was a vile tyrant, a murderer, an oppressor of his subjects, he bought up all commodities, and sold them at his own price, sold abbeys to Jews and Falkoners; both Ferdinand his father, and he himself never made conscience of any committed sin; and to conclude, saith he, it was impossible to do worse than they did. Why was Pausanias the Spartan tyrant,

Nero, Otho, Galba, so persecuted with spirits in every house they came, but for their murders which they had committed? Why doth the devil haunt many men's houses after their deaths, appear to them living, and take possession of their habitations, as it were, of their palaces, but because of their several villainies? Yea, and sometimes GOD himself hath a hand in it, to show his power, humiliate, exercise, and to try their faith . . . God the avenger . . .'.

My tentative suggestion is that Keats thought this might make a good plot for a play. His curious and undatable fragment, 'This living hand . . .' has been thought by several editors to be intended for a play, and its tone and theme accord with Burton's example of the conscience-stricken Alphonsus, whose revenant father had died of grief for his son's sins:

This living hand, now warm and capable
Of earnest grasping, would, if it were cold
And in the icy silence of the tomb,
So haunt thy days and chill thy dreaming nights
That thou would wish thine own heart dry of blood
So in my veins red life might stream again,
And thou be conscience-calmed – see here it is –
I hold it towards you.

The subject itself would also have appealed to Keats's interest in remorseful tyrants in relation to the Hyperion project. His indignation against bullies and tyrannical behaviour had been a characteristic evident since school days, and activated at various periods when he encountered it, as when his friend Bailey was treated shoddily by the Bishop of Lincoln in 1817. Modern historians confirm Burton's account of the fate of 'Alfonso of Aragon, King of Naples', whose kingdom was invaded by Charles, King of France. Facing defeat, Alfonso was warned by his doctor that a ghost of one of Alfonso's victims had appeared in a dream threatening a bad end for him, so Alfonso abdicated and fled to a monastery.[65] 'This living hand . . .' again seems pertinent as an appeal to remorse. If Keats did indeed see dramatic potential in this plot, he has not been alone. As a tantalising postscript, Alfonso has indeed been portrayed dramatically, twice in fact: in 2011 in the BBC television series *The Borgias* and in the 2013 series depicting a fictional account of Leonardo's early life, *Da Vinci's Demons*, again from the BBC.

The final page indexed by Keats most obviously bears out the hypothesis that he is listing sections in Burton which may have offered possible subjects for his own works. It reads '197 Lamia. Part 3. Memb. 1st. Subs. I.'. Beside the passage in the text is a pencilled note, presumably by Brown, reading 'Keats Lamia'. Some implications for Keats's poem will be discussed in Chapter 6. Beside Burton's phrase 'vanished in an instant'

Keats placed a cross and wrote, 'and was never after seen'. In 'Lamia' this becomes 'no sooner said, | Than with a frightful scream she vanished'. There is then another pencilled note here, 'Hunt's Indicator', no doubt Brown's reference to Hunt's approval of Keats's poem in his review of the volume. At least here in the last item listed in Keats's 'index' we are on firm ground, knowing that Burton was indeed the source for a poem. For the others, clear explanations are not forthcoming, though it does seem that they deal with lovers and tyrants, reminding us of Bottom's taste in *A Midsummer Night's Dream*: '. . . my chief humour is for a tyrant. I could play Ercles rarely, or a part to tear a cat in, to make all split . . . This is Ercles' vein, a tyrant's vein; a lover is more condoling' (1.2.25–38 *passim*). Except that Burton's lovers are generally far from 'condoling'.

By way of conclusion, we might say that what distinguishes Burton from those who had written before him on melancholy is the extraordinarily wide ambit he gives to the condition. Whereas others had written serious accounts in sustained, scholarly mode of the malady marked by fear and sorrow without reason or cause, he includes in its orbit virtually everything under the sun relating to emotional aberrancies, all described in a dazzling array of styles and tones. It was undoubtedly the book's extraordinary inclusiveness and intellectual range that appealed to Keats, since his markings draw out and display these aspects. Burton's book is also a study which is of special significance to writers, to the extent that he presents melancholy as quintessentially a writer's way of seeing the world, turning life into art and applying fiction to life. As one scholar has put it,

> This was more than a treatise about the black bile that caused or was correlated with melancholy; Burton had written a paean to the literary, mythological, historical , and philosophical richness of the states that melancholy named . . . it remains a veritable encyclopedia of everything there was to know, at the time, that could conceivably have anything to do with the melancholic condition – or indeed with the human condition. As Burton put it, '[T]he tower of Babel never yielded such confusion of tongues, as the chaos of melancholy doth variety of symptoms' . . .[66]

Considerably briefer in length, but in its own way just as ambitious as Burton's tome in its emotional range, was Keats's poetic enterprise in 1819. While revelling in the words and spirit of *The Anatomy*, he was writing and collecting poems for a poetic 'paean' to melancholy in all its diversity, *Lamia, Isabella, The Eve of St Agnes, and Other Poems*. This was his own 'anatomy of melancholy': 'Ay, in the very temple of Delight | Veil'd Melancholy has her sacred shrine'. To his own poems we now turn.

Notes

1. See Keats, *The Complete Works of John Keats*, ed. H. Buxton Forman, 3, p. 306.
2. An argument for a later date, April 1819, is advanced by Sinson, p. 14.
3. To George and Georgiana Keats 17–27 September 1819. *LJK* 2, p. 192.
4. *KC*, 1, p. 254.
5. See Gittings, *John Keats: The Living Year*, 'Appendix A: Parallels Between Burton's *Anatomy of Melancholy* and Keats's Poems and Letters', pp. 215–18.
6. Jack, p. 37.
7. *KC*, 1, 260, fn.
8. Keats, *The Complete Works*, ed. H. Buxton Forman, 3, pp. 306–20.
9. *KC*, 1, p. 258. On Keats's library see Brown's listing in *KC* 1, pp. 253–60; Owings, *The Keats Library: A Descriptive Catalogue*; and the more analytical study by Lau, 'Analyzing Keats's Library by Genre'.
10. References in vol. 1 are to the standard editions, while in the volume owned by Keats I quote page numbers from that volume, now in Keats House in Hampstead. For convenience, I have quoted from the 'Gutenberg Project' online edition, transcribed (and occasionally corrected) from the 1813 edition read by Keats, itself a modernised version of the latest seventeenth century edition. Also available is a digital facsimile of Volume 2 on the Internet Archive (1821), a reprint of 1813: <https://archive.org/stream/b29328433_0002?ref=ol#page/n6/mode/2up> (last accessed 20 March 2020). For the rhetorical background with which Burton is here associating and distancing himself, see Gowland, 'Rhetorical Structure and Function in *The Anatomy of Melancholy*'.
11. To Reynolds, 3 May, 1818, *LJK*, 1, p. 279.
12. Tompkins, p. 225 and *passim*.
13. McQuillan, p. 139. See also Tompkins, *Reader-Response Criticism*.
14. Iser, *The Act of Reading: A Theory of Aesthetic Response*; Holland, *5 Readers Reading*; Jauss, *Toward an Aesthetic of Reception*.
15. Barthes had used the phrase in several essays from 1967 onwards, and in his book, *Image-Music-Text*. See also Barthes, *S / Z*.
16. See Stockwell, ch. 5, 'Identification and Resistance'.
17. Falkes, pp. 47–59. On the general subject, see also Ou, *Keats and Negative Capability*.
18. To George and Tom Keats, 21 December, 1817, *LJK* 1, p. 193.
19. He is bringing to bear upon a text and also revealing his own 'experiential knowledge' in the company of books. Charles Cowden Clarke, p. 120.
20. For more detailed analysis of the process, see R. S. White, *Keats as a Reader of Shakespeare*, ch. 1, and Lau, 'John Keats' pp. 109–59.
21. Lau, *Keats's Paradise Lost*, p. 68.
22. The reference is to Spurgeon, *Keats's Shakespeare: A Descriptive Study*.
23. To George and Georgina Keats, 21 September 1819, *LJK, 2*, p. 213.
24. To Woodhouse, 27 October 1818, *LJK, 1*, p. 387.
25. Reference Bodleian 2698 e.58 (v. 2).

26. See Keymer, pp. 153–4.
27. Ferriar, *Illustrations of Sterne with Other Essays and Verses*. I am very grateful to Jon Mee for drawing to my attention this fascinating work.
28. Read, p. 330, footnoted by New, p. 135.
29. *OED*.
30. One hypothetical candidate that occurs to me is that George may be a sibling of John Taylor, Keats's publisher, who was the third of nine children in an evidently erudite family. Nicholas Roe (doyen among biographers) suggests in correspondence: 'I had a look at George Taylors in *Alumni Oxoniensis 1715–1886*: there are a dozen of them (I expected more) and most of them are obviously not your George Taylor. However, one of them, fifth down in the right-hand column on p. 1393 is at least a possibility. BA Pembroke Cambridge 1815, MA 1821, DCL St John's Oxford 1827, later Rector and 'Lecturer' of Dedham in Essex: <http://www.historyhouse. co.uk/placeD/essexd08d.html> (last accessed 20 March 2020).
31. See Burton, 'Marginalia in Burton's *The Art of Melancholy*, Royal College of Physicians of Edinburgh <http://www.rcpe.ac.uk/heritage/marginalia-burtons-anatomy-melancholy-1821> (last accessed 20 March 2020).
32. To the George Keatses, 18 September 1819, *LJK*, 2, pp. 192–3.
33. O'Neill, p. 103.
34. *OED* (1) and (2). Keats had used it to describe Hazlitt's excoriating, public 'Letter to Gifford' quoted at length in To the George Keatses, 12 March 1819, *LJK*, 2, p. 73.
35. Ward, p. 544.
36. Hessell, p. 96.
37. For details see Evans, 'Poison Wine', p. 35.
38. For suggestions on the plants sketched and their possible significance, see Evans, 'Nice Ink, Keats. The medical student and his botanicall literary doodle'.
39. Motion, p. 364.
40. Ward, p. 548.
41. Bamborough, p. xxv.
42. To Reynolds, 11, 13 July 1818, *LJK*, 1, p. 324.
43. See Davies, 'Keats's Killing Breath: Paradigms of a Pathology'. See also Goellnicht, pp. 194–8.
44. Bari, ch. 3.
45. Murray,1, p. 355.
46. de Almeida, *Romantic Medicine*, p. 166.
47. *The Fall of Hyperion*, Canto 1, p. 190.
48. To Bailey, 14 August 1819, *LJK*, 2, p. 139.
49. Gittings, *The Living Year*, p. 52.
50. 'John Hatfield' in *Oxford Dictionary of National Biography*.
51. Sinson, pp. 17–18.
52. Quoted Sinson, 19, from Burton Part 1, Sect. 3, Mem. 1. Subs. 1, 455 in 1813 edn; and Part 1, Sect. 3, Mem. 1. Subs. 2, 459 in 1813 edition.
53. To Fanny Brawne 15(?) July, 1819, *LJK*, 2, p. 130. Rollins identifies the tale as coming from Henry Weber's *Tales of the East* (1812).
54. Spenser, *The Faerie Queene*, 1.9.13–16.
55. See especially Homans, 'Keats Reading Women, Women Reading Keats';

Wolfson, "Feminizing Keats" and 'Keats's "Gordian Complication" of Women'; Arseneau, Madeline, Mermaids, and Medusas in "The Eve of St Agnes"'; Mellor, 'Keats and the Complexities of Gender'.

56. To the George Keatses, 14–31 October 1818, *LJK*, 1, pp. 395–6.
57. *LJK*, 1, 395; 2, p. 133.
58. To Bailey 18 July, 1818, *LJK*, 1, p. 341.
59. Ibid. pp. 341–2.
60. Arseneau, p. 235.
61. Stillinger, *The Poems of John Keats*, p. 645.
62. Gittings, *John Keats: The Living Year*, p. 117.
63. Whale, p. 23.
64. Schulkins, p. 111, cf. p. 67.
65. Hersey, p. 6.
66. Arikha, p. 141.

CONTENTS.

———

6.1 Image of the 1820 Contents page, The British Library, shelfmark C.39.b.67. In the public domain.

Chapter 6

'Moods of My Own Mind': Keats's Anatomy of Melancholy. The Poems

'Lamia'

We know there was discussion between poet and publishers concerning which poem should open *1820*, but not why 'Lamia' emerged as front-runner. Of the longer poems, 'The Eve of St. Agnes', which was Keats's initial choice, has been more kindly treated by posterity. 'Lamia' was one work which Keats seemed satisfied with, writing of it to Reynolds, 'I make use of my Judgment more deliberately than I yet have done',[1] but this may not be enough as an explanation. Being the latest of the three longer poems, written between June and September 1819 (finished just before 'To Autumn' on 22 September), Keats may have thought it his most mature and up to date. However, it is significant that 'Lamia' explicitly references the book which has been his companion during 1819, Burton's *The Anatomy of Melancholy*, and it also begins the volume's internal debate, beginning with Burton's leading concept of 'heroical love melancholy' treated in its various guises. (The term should have been 'erotic love' since 'heroical' was a medieval misunderstanding of Greek 'eros' for 'hereos' dating back to a mistranslation in Chaucer's *The Knight's Tale*, but its currency persisted through to Burton's time.)[2] Its placement at the start of the volume explicitly signals that not only is the plot taken from Burton, but also something of *The Anatomy of Melancholy* will be thematically present in the volume as a whole, since that work provides the only footnote in the book. In a thorough and suggestive essay from which I draw, Jane Chambers acknowledges the pervasive debt, though restricting her account to 'Lamia' alone: 'A journey through *Lamia* with Robert Burton as our guide will illustrate the value of such a source study', revealing more than just the narrative.[3] Partially excepting only Charles I. Patterson in *The Daemonic in the Poetry of John Keats*,[4] Chambers notices with irony that, for other scholars, 'seeking literary sources *except* Burton is important'.[5]

Keats found some information about *lamiae* in his indispensable copy of Lemprière's *Classical Dictionary*. This offers the information that they were monsters from Africa who had 'the face and breast of a woman, and the rest of the body like a serpent', and that their 'pleasant and agreeable' hissing lured people, especially children, whom they promptly paralysed and devoured.[6] However, Keats's transcription of a whole passage in the footnote after the poem establishes that *The Anatomy of Melancholy* was his primary source. His own poetic narrative is considerably more sympathetic to the character than Lemprière's account, since Keats follows Burton in allowing her to have an ambiguous emotional life. In his copy of Burton's book, Keats has solidly side-marked a passage, emphasising by underlining a phrase within it:

> I know that Biarmannus ... and some others <u>stoutly deny it</u>, *that the devil hath any carnal copulation with women, that the devil takes no pleasure in such facts, they be mere fantasies, all such relations of incubi, succubi, lies and tales;* ... *but* ... (pp. 195–6)

This leads on to the quotation which Keats supplies in his footnote, transcribed complete with the scholarly reference to the passage in Burton, as follows:

> Philostratus, in his fourth book *De Vita Apollonii,* hath a memorable instance in this kind, which I may not omit, of one Menippus Lycius, a young man twenty five years of age, that going betwixt Cenchreas and Corinth, met such a phantasm in the habit of a fair gentlewoman, which taking him by the hand, carried him home to her house, in the suburbs of Corinth, and told him she was a Phoenician by birth, and if he would tarry with her, he should hear her sing and play, and drink such wine as never any drank, and no man should molest him; but she, being fair and lovely, would live and die with him, that was fair and lovely to behold. The young man, a philosopher, otherwise staid and discreet, able to moderate his passions, though not this of love, tarried with her a while to his great content, and at last married her, to whose wedding, amongst other guests, came Apollonius; who, by some probable conjectures, found her out to be a serpent, a lamia; and that all her furniture was, like Tantalus' gold, described by Homer, no substance but mere illusions. When she saw herself descried, she wept, and desired Apollonius to be silent, but he would not be moved, and thereupon she, plate, house, and all that was in it, vanished in an instant: many thousands took notice of this fact, for it was done in the midst of Greece.
>
> Burton's 'Anatomy of Melancholy.' *Part 3. Sect. 2. Memb. 1. Subs. 1*

Sperry suggests that 'the very vulnerability and lack of depth of Burton's characters constituted a positive asset' since it allowed Keats free rein to flesh out the details and, importantly, to maintain an ambivalence 'with a deliberate irony of stance and manner'.[7] Keats shifts the points of view between Lamia, Lycius and Apollonius, whereas Burton's attention is limited to the lamia's feelings, in illustrating his own chosen subject of devils or other immortals falling in love with mortals. (This had, of course, been the central premise of *Endymion* so it interested Keats, even if he may not yet have read Burton when he wrote that poem.) Moreover, Keats also employs different aspects of the Burtonian world view and style.

In Chapter 3, I suggested the importance of eyes in the imagery of this poem and others in Keats's volume, and in this light it seems significant that he introduces Lamia in her serpent state as being a 'beautiful wreath with melancholy eyes', weeping for her own pitiable solitude to which she is condemned so long as she remains trapped in serpent form. To change into a human form she needs the help of shape-changing Hermes, 'the only sad one' among the gods, frustrated as he is himself and 'bent on amorous theft'. He is marked as a false healer, carrying a 'serpent rod' (caduceus), but showing two twined serpents rather than the one signifying Aesculapius the true healer.[8] He is useful to Lamia since he can make dreams come true, and she strikes a bargain with him that she can find his desired 'wood-nymph' in return for her transformation. Both represent the kind of obsessional love-melancholy which is Burton's subject in this section of the *Anatomy*, demonstrating that even nonhumans can be afflicted by this nonrational and distressing emotional state. At this stage Keats, like Burton, maintains narratorial inwardness with Lamia's consciousness, drawing the reader's sympathy as she suffers the symptoms, since she has already fallen helplessly in love on seeing the Corinthian youth Lycius.

The perspective changes to external observation. Even in its ugliness, the lamia as 'palpitating' snake has a paradoxical aesthetic fascination, which Keats as poet demonstrates in a passage exemplifying Hazlitt's 'gusto', defined as 'power or passion defining any object . . . some precise association with pleasure or pain':[9]

> She was a Gordian shape of dazzling hue,
>
> *
>
> Vermilion-spotted, golden, green, and blue;
> So rainbow-sided, touch'd with miseries,
> She seem'd, at once, some penanced lady elf,
> Some demon's mistress, or the demon's self.

Described as 'bitter-sweet' in appearance, Lamia's painful moment of transition is presented as a literal shedding of the snake's dazzling colours

– 'She writh'd about, convuls'd with scarlet pain' – until 'Nothing but pain and ugliness were left'; whereupon she vanishes and reappears as 'now a lady bright, I A full-blown beauty new and exquisite . . .'. Such collocations of beauty and ugliness, pain and pleasure, darkness and light, fair and foul, are typical of Keats's poetry and letters, a part of his temperamental signature. This he found also in Burton: *'our whole life is a perpetual combat, a conflict, a set battle, a snarling fit'* (p. 184, side-marked). Such paradoxes abound, especially when he is speaking of love, often drawing on standard Platonic explanations:

> Ficinus, in his comment upon this place, *cap. 8.* following Plato, calls these two loves, two devils, or good and bad angels according to us, which are still hovering about our souls. "The one rears to heaven, the other depresseth us to hell; the one good, which stirs us up to the contemplation of that divine beauty for whose sake we perform justice and all godly offices, study philosophy, &c.; the other base, and though bad yet to be respected; for indeed both are good in their own natures . . ." (p. 162, not marked)

For Burton, the doubleness of love has a physiological basis:

> The rational resides in the brain, the other in the liver (as before hath been said out of Plato and others); the heart is diversely affected of both, and carried a thousand ways by consent. The sensitive faculty most part overrules reason, the soul is carried hoodwinked, and the understanding captive like a beast. "The heart is variously inclined, sometimes they are merry, sometimes sad, and from love arise hope and fear, jealousy, fury, desperation." (p. 167; not marked, but close to Keats's note on 'the old plague spot': see above)

(We notice, by the way, that the loaded word 'hoodwinked' occurs in 'The Eve of St Agnes'.) In 'Lamia' the contradictions between appearance and reality, and the bewildering visual changes, become analogues for love itself in a Burtonian sense. Lamia knows Lycius would be filled with fear and loathing should he witness her reptilian state, while her desire to change appearance is in order to gain access to his company and elicit his love. Her metamorphosed, pseudohuman image is named as a 'dream', an illusion:

> And sometimes into cities she would send
> Her dream, with feast and rioting to blend;
> And once, while among mortals dreaming thus,
> She saw the young Corinthian Lycius.

Her knowledge of love is as contradictory and complex as Burton's representation of erotic love:

> A virgin purest lipp'd, yet in the lore
> Of love deep learned to the red heart's core:

Not one hour old, yet of sciential brain
To unperplex bliss from its neighbour pain.

Burton had generalised that love is a form of witchcraft operating through eyesight, another hint picked up by Keats:

> Now last of all, I will show you by what means beauty doth fascinate, bewitch, as some hold, and work upon the soul of a man by the eye. For certainly I am of the poet's mind, love doth bewitch and strangely change us.
>> Love mocks our senses, curbs our liberties,
>> And doth bewitch us with his art and rings,
>> I think some devil gets into our entrails,
>> And kindles coals, and heaves our souls from th'hinges.
>
> Heliodorus lib. 3. proves at large, that love is witchcraft, "it gets in at our eyes, pores, nostrils, engenders the same qualities and affections in us, as were in the party whence it came." The manner of the fascination, as Ficinus 10. cap. com. in Plat. declares it, is thus: "Mortal men are then especially bewitched, when as by often gazing one on the other, they direct sight to sight, join eye to eye, and so drink and suck in love between them; for the beginning of this disease is the eye . . ."
>
> (Book III, Memb II, Subsect. II, not marked)

After the transformation, the point of view is sympathetically aligned with Lamia's consciousness as she falls into 'a swooning love' of Lycius, building up a reservoir of pity for her which will inform the ending of the poem. As in Shakespeare's *Venus and Adonis*, an immortal's love for a mortal is doomed because each exists in different time dimensions, and that which never dies cannot sustain a relationship with one who does. In *Endymion* Keats had resolved the problem by fusing the goddess Cynthia and the Indian maid into a single earthly figure, but Lamia's fundamental, immortal identity as serpent prevents such an easy solution since it depends on deception and disguise. Anticipating their inevitable mutual suffering, the imagery, tone and perspective rather suddenly switch again when Lycius falls in love with her, as she is now viewed unsympathetically from the outside: 'The cruel lady, without any show | Of sorrow for her tender favourite's woe . . . The life she had so tangled in her mesh'. Fast upon deception come her strategic lies about her pretended, secluded life in Corinth. She is, in calculated fashion, 'playing woman's part', casting 'a spell' upon the 'blinded' Lycius. He is now cast as unwitting victim, 'and he never thought to know'. A touch of Burton's habit of seeing female beauty as untrustworthy and potentially fatal has crept into the poem's frame. Lycius's love is stirred at first sight and sound of the weeping, inadvertently seductive, 'enticing' figure:

Lycius from death awoke into amaze,
To see her still, and singing so sweet lays;

Then from amaze into delight he fell
To hear her whisper woman's lore so well;
And every word she spake entic'd him on
To unperplex'd delight and pleasure known.

From Lamia's love-melancholy, experienced as erotic frustration, the poem now moves on to love-melancholy of Lycius in his deluded blindness. Each type – deceiver and deceived – has its place in Burton's taxonomy of love. At this stage Apollonius passes by, 'robed in philosophic gown', chilling Lamia and causing Lycius to hide himself 'from his quick eyes' as though from embarrassment at being seen with a woman by his tutor.

The switches of tone at the end of Part I and beginning of Part II are also reminiscent of the aspects of Burton's style and viewpoint which had attracted Keats. Verbal playfulness and ironic detachment creep into the narrator's stance:

Let the mad poets say whate'er they please
Of the sweets of Fairies, Paris, Goddesses,
There is not such a treat among them all,
Haunters of cavern, lake and waterfall,
As a real woman . . .

There are multiple ironies, first at the expense of 'mad poets' extolling immortals while ignoring human beings, and secondly because Lamia is, of course, not a 'real woman' but a fairy, demon, or even goddess. Thirdly, irony is angled at the poet-narrator here, since he is indulging the kind of fiction which the poetry itself now reproves, showing that the beauty of a 'real woman' may be only an appearance based on poetic deception and embellishment. Such ironies occur often in Burton's *Anatomy*, for example, in his account of the lamia itself in which he claims not to believe in what he yet still goes on to retell. They are also characteristic of Keats's own conflicted and fluctuating attitudes to women as goddesses and temptresses. The same undercutting playfulness underlies the ending of Part I:

But the flitter-winged verse must tell,
For truth's sake, what woe afterwards befell,
'Twould humour many a heart to leave them thus,
Shut from the busy world of more incredulous.

Jane Chambers cites with approval the few critics who have detected notes of humour,[10] at least in the first half of the poem, and she chooses to find its source in 'the humorous undertone of the entire *Anatomy* . . .'.[11] Of these critics, Georgia S. Dunbar finds a sustained 'charming good humor' in the first half of Keats's poem, especially in the early section with Hermes, to be 'replaced by a very different kind of mockery – satire and sarcasm' in the second.[12] This may overstate the case since any hint of 'satire and sarcasm' is tempered by sympathy for the pained vulnerability of Lamia in particular, and the later feelings of Lycius. What seems more to the point – and more like Burton – is the rapid switching of tones, never allowing one mood, whether serious or lighthearted, to settle into a norm. Emotional investment is punctured by rational detachment, in both 'Lamia' and Burton's *Anatomy*.

This is especially evident in the jocularly expressed opening lines of Part II: 'Love in a hut, with water and a crust, | Is – Love forgive us! – cinders, ashes, dust'. The intrusive thought seems to have a Burtonian edge in the digressive, debunking detachment and wry sententiousness, stylistic facets which Keats had relished in his reading of the *Anatomy*. The sentiment itself is also of dubious relevance at this point in the poem and may even be Keats's sardonic reflection on his own bleak amatory prospects at the time when it was written. He was facing considerable pecuniary difficulties, fuelling Mrs Brawne's reservations about wedding her daughter into such a financially insecure plight. The abruptly inter-polated thought provides another, sudden shift of perspective, preparing for the ending by redirecting attention away from the lovers' feelings to love itself as based on fantasy or illusion, eventually to be destroyed by the intrusion of a more brutally unillusioned gaze. As Burton had implied in his commentary, the lamia is probably another example of the opinion that, *'they be mere fantasies, all such relations of incubi, succubi, lies and tales'*. Remember his mischievous joke that idealising a lover may be just another fantasy: 'anyone who loves a frog thinks that frog to be Diana'? This is the troubling conclusion towards which Keats's poem now heads, prefaced by the lines following the 'Love in a hut' couplet:

Love in a palace is perhaps at last
More grievous torment than a hermit's fast: –
That is a doubtful tale from faery land,
Hard for the non-elect to understand.

First, however, the mood changes again from satirical detachment back to emotional sympathy. The narrative is relocated in Lamia's anxious mind and her 'grievous torment' in realising that the lovers' sequestered privacy must end. They must emerge from their secluded 'purple-lined palace of sweet sin' to undergo what, for her, is a terrible ordeal. Lycius notices her new, melancholy 'sad forlorn' state and he is now the one labelled 'cruel': 'Against his better self, he took delight | Luxurious in her sorrows, soft and new'. Her distress is palpable as she 'wept a rain | Of sorrows at his words'. She reluctantly agrees to Lycius's request for the public celebration of a wedding, but repeats her darkest fear in the request, '"Old Apollonius – from him keep me hid"'. In the third occurrence of the word in the poem, Lycius is 'perplex'd', a particular favourite of Burton's since he repeats it seventeen times in the *Anatomy*, usually in groups such as 'full of perplexity, danger, and misery' and 'perplexities and cares'. As the celebration is prepared, Lamia silently paces around in a conflicted mood of generalised melancholy, 'In pale contented sort of discontent'. The narrator steps in to issue a strong warning which is unheeded:

> 'O senseless Lycius! Madman! Wherefore flout
> The silent-blessing fate, warm and cloister'd hours,
> And show to common eyes those secret bowers?

Choose to remain in a state of blissful blindness and the poet's fantasy, he seems to suggest, and do not risk reality intruding to break the spell.

The point of view rapidly shifts now from emotional quandary to hard-edged humour, as the wedding guests are seen as a 'herd' marvelling at the palace's opulence. Once again to Lycius's embarrassment (he blushes), Apollonius arrives as 'uninvited guest' 'with eye severe', and he laughs enigmatically to himself as though he has solved 'some knotty problem'. The party seems to go well. The guests become increasingly drunk as 'the happy vintage touch'd their brains' and even the verse seems to become tipsily descriptive, 'for merry wine, sweet wine, | Will make Elysian shades not too fair, too divine'. All are garlanded with a plant wreath individualised 'to suit the thought | Of every guest', revealing a range of moods, reminiscent of Burton's botanical lore. On the 'aching head' of Lamia is placed 'The leaves of willow and of adder's tongue'. Willow is associated with 'weeping' and adder's tongue is a plant named for its appearance as a serpent's tongue. On Lycius is placed the thyrsus (Bacchus's wand, twined with ivy and vine leaves), linking him with drunken lack of perceptiveness, 'that his watching eyes may swim | Into forgetfulness'. To Apollonius is given 'spear-grass and the spiteful thistle', whose spiky, hostile associations are evident in the words. The 'bald-head philosopher' brings the festivities to an uncomfortably abrupt termination with his exposure: '"Begone, foul dream!"' he exclaims to Lamia, and to Lycius, '"And shall I see thee made a serpent's prey?"'. Lamia disappears 'with a frightful scream', and Lycius immediately dies: 'And in its marriage robe, the heavy body wound'. In this, the first poem in the collection, Lycius has become the first of those mentioned in the last, 'Ode on Melancholy', as one who is

Melancholy's victim and is 'among her cloudy trophies hung'.[13] He is to be joined by Isabella, the Beadsman and Angela in 'The Eve of St Agnes', and finally the poet himself.

The significance of the narrator's comment on Apollonius's intervention has been debated and variously defined by critics. Andrew Bennett, for example, suggests various correspondences, including the sceptical Charles Brown and the baleful reviewers who had attempted to destroy Keats's earlier published poems.[14] But generally Apollonius is seen to be associated with science in opposition to the mysteries of poetry. The poem itself challenges the 'cold philosophy' of the scientific method (known at the time as 'natural philosophy'):

> Do not all charms fly
> At the mere touch of cold philosophy?
> There was an awful rainbow once in heaven:
> We know her woof, her texture; she is given
> In the dull catalogue of common things.
> Philosophy will clip an Angel's wings,
> Conquer all mysteries by rule and line,
> Empty the haunted air, and gnomed mine –
> Unweave a rainbow, as it erewhile made
> The tender-person'd Lamia melt into a shade.

The usual references offered for these lines are first to Hazlitt's lecture, 'On Poetry in General' (1818): 'It cannot be concealed that ... the progress of knowledge and refinement has a tendency to circumscribe the limits of the imagination, and to clip the wings of poetry',[15] and secondly to Keats's agreement with Lamb's provocation at a dinner-party at Haydon's on 28 December, 1817, in claiming that Newton had 'destroyed all the Poetry of the rainbow, by reducing it to a prism', going on to drink to 'Newton's health, and confusion to mathematics'.[16] Keats repeated a similar scepticism about his age's sensibility, in his review in *The Champion*, 21 December, 1817 of Kean's acting: 'In our unimaginative days – *Habeas Corpus'd* as we are, out of all wonder, uncertainty and fear ...'.[17] It is plausible that he also had in mind the mauling his own two earlier volumes of poetry had received from the 'Keen, cruel, perceant, stinging' reviewers.

The spirit of these multiple references does lie behind the passage in 'Lamia' and they would support a reading resting on the poet's disappointment in the kind of rationalistic, post-Newtonian scientific analysis which destroys the beautiful illusions of poetry. However, other experiential sources occur which complicate the context, and they go to the heart of the melancholy that pervades the poem. The first is Keats's experiences of medicine in Guy's Hospital, when he observed at first hand the dismaying truths about the frail and too-easily destructible human body. He had witnessed it on a daily basis, in the beds and on the anatomy slab, beauty reduced to physical decay, and as Nicholas Roe observes, he had himself 'dissected corpses in various multi-coloured states of nauseating decomposition'.[18] A similar experience seems to have been in his mind later when, watching his brother Tom dying, he wrote to Bailey sharing the different sources of their 'discontented nerves'– Bailey's due to credulity, his own to a sceptical, untrusting doubt – when he concludes, 'were it in my choice I would reject a petrarchal coronation – on account of my dying day, and because Women have cancers'.[19] Here he casts Bailey in the position of the optimistic and deluded Lycius, and himself as having been trained into realistic observation of the discrepancy between the human body alive and dead. Apollonius then becomes a kind of Astley Cooper figure, healing while necessarily causing pain, with an unflinching suppression of sympathetic identification with his suffering patients in the interests of humanitarian efficiency in his profession. A fatalistic and ultimately necessary realism, then, motivates the philosopher, since Lycius cannot live forever in illusion, just as Lamia cannot forever sustain the illusion of being a woman. That Apollonius inadvertently causes the death of the 'patient', Lycius, must also have been a frequent occurrence at Guy's. The diagnosis at the end – 'no pulse, or breath they found' in the 'heavy body' – evokes this sobering medical ambience.

The second reference is to Keats's other 'tutor' in philosophy, Robert Burton, who also, incidentally, refers to the way Cupid 'had his wings clipped' by the council of gods, 'that he might come no more among them' (p. 192). In *The Anatomy of Melancholy* Burton manages, sometimes alternately and sometimes simultaneously, to idealise and undercut both love and beauty. He trains the Keatsian reader into a habit of believing and yet not believing in the life-enhancing qualities of the doomed illusions that poets depend on. Burton's narrator in the first section, Democritus Junior, insists that the only reasonable response to love is both to laugh and cry in the face of a power which 'can make mad and sober whom he list . . . can make sick and cure whom he list'.[20] Ambivalent to the end, 'Lamia' leaves open various possibilities about the dispersal of sympathies between the figures, and poses moral questions about whether it is merciful or merciless to maintain an illusion or puncture it. Such ruminations raised by the melancholy mind persist through Keats's collection in a variety of presentations. 'Lamia' sets up a series of polarities between beauty and truth, illusion and reality, ecstasy and agony, and it questions whether love and beauty can coexist with open-eyed observation of reality. Subsequent poems play variations upon, and seek to reconcile such contradictions, moving towards a position that places the poet as one who can heal emotional wounds and offer different forms of consolation for loss and melancholy.

More generally, 'Lamia' shows links between Burton's and Keats's respective and reductive views of women addressed in Chapter 5. In terms of literary influences, Burton certainly aided and abetted the divided and suspicious view of women, but in Keats's earlier reading, *The Faerie Queene* also provided a poetic precedent. Spenser's women divide between the holiness of Una on the one hand, and on the other the deceiving Duessa, enchantress and *femme fatale*:

> Her nether parts misshapen, monstruous,
> Were hidd in water, that I could not see,
> But they did seeme more foule and hideous,
> Then womans shape man would beleeve to bee.
>
> (1.2.41–4)

The more unsympathetic aspects of Lamia, and the near-monstrosity of the love depicted, contain an element of the repulsion behind Keats's 'the old scrofula' annotation.

Overall, it is Burton who presides over 'Lamia', providing the basis of the story, a narrative stance constantly switching between detachment and sympathy, painful perplexities created when the immortal intersects with the mortal condition, unexpected juxtapositions of humour and tragedy, beauty and ugliness, conflicted attitudes towards women, and ineffectual resistance to the melancholy realisation that love engendered through the eyes and based on physical beauty alone, is unlikely to survive the piercing acuity of reason or pressures of reality. In Keats's volume, vestiges and variations of such 'perplexities' are reflected in other poems, and 'Lamia' stands as a conceptual portal to the collection.

'Isabella; or, The Pot of Basil'

'Isabella', headlined in *1820* as 'A STORY FROM BOCCACCIO', may contain fewer direct links with *The Anatomy of Melancholy* than 'Lamia', but its subject matter and prevailing worldview overlap just as much with Burton's quasi-medical approach to love and melancholy. The poem's composition between February and April, 1818 predated Keats's saturation in Burton's *Anatomy* during 1819, though this does not necessarily mean he had not already read the book. In fact, some of the quotations below might begin a case that he had read it, but the medical knowledge Burton draws on would have been generally available to Keats from other sources and from his own training. At the very least it shows a predisposition in Keats to leap upon Burton as a fellow spirit. There are in the poem both latent and blatant medical references, and the deteriorating emotional and physical state of Isabella is pathologised in almost clinical fashion as a classic case of melancholy. As in 'Lamia' there are signs once again that Keats was recalling his reading in medicine, to the extent that 'Isabella' is his most iatric work. He draws, for example, on the 'like cures like' theory of sympathetic medicine, that symptoms caused by a particular substance can be cured by controlled, minimal doses of the same substance: 'Even bees, the little almsmen of spring-bowers, | Know there is richest juice in poison-flowers' (Stanza XIII), the last phrase resembling Astley Cooper's 'all poisonous substances in small doses can be beneficial medicines'.[21] By including different states of melancholy in 'Isabella', Keats turns Boccaccio's story into a clinically focused study. Hermione de Almeida writes, 'With typical Keatsian but also pharmacological reciprocity, the poem *Isabella: Or, the Pot of Basil* bears illness as its dominant metaphor even as its subject, or essence, is love'.[22]

Just as significant as the medical background is the literary context. The poem had been intended as a contribution to a collaborative project with John Hamilton Reynolds, to versify tales from Boccaccio, along the lines of Reynolds' own works published in *The Garden of Florence: and Other Poems* (1821). The suggestion had come in a lecture by Hazlitt which Keats attended on 3 February 1818.[23] In addition, the Della Cruscan fashion for verse translations from Renaissance Italian writers had not entirely run its course, and 'Barry Cornwall' was writing similar adaptations, such as *A Sicilian Story*, also based on Boccaccio.[24] Shelley enthusiastically endorsed Boccaccio as being politically compatible with the views of Hunt's 'Cockney School', and Coleridge too was an admirer.[25] In other words, 'Isabella' was written within a contemporary literary culture which included also the Gothic revival and the tail-end of the vogue for graveyard poetry. However, Keats makes the territory his own by amplifying melancholy as a medical and psychological condition, compared with Boccaccio's very sketchy account. Melancholy is at the heart of Keats's 'Isabella; or, the Pot of Basil'.

Although lacking the Burtonian stylistic elements evident in 'Lamia'– switching perspectives, digressiveness, jokes, irony and satire, all mingled with sympathy for suffering protagonists – nonetheless 'Isabella' is a sustained 'case study' of melancholy, taking us into some of the darkest sides of the condition. The world it presents is Burton's. In particular, there are two separate forms depicted. The first is love-melancholy, which could be cured most effectively in Burton's eyes by mutually fulfilled love. The symptomatic physiology is evident in the early stages of the poem. Isabella and Lorenzo both 'nightly weep' (I); he is insomniac with 'sick longing' (III), and both are in a 'sad plight' which makes 'their cheeks paler' (IV). The condition is especially noticeable in Isabella, whose suffering is clear from her bodily reactions, as Lorenzo observes:

> "How ill she is," said he, "I may not speak,
> "And yet I will, and tell my love all plain:
> "If looks speak love-laws, I will drink her tears,
> "And at the least 'twill startle off her cares."
>
> (V)

Similar signs are also evident in his own bodily state, as 'his heart beat awfully against his side', he is tongue-tied and 'fever'd' (VI), and Isabella notices his forehead 'waxing very pale and dead' (VII). Burton had written,

> *Shall I say, most part of a lover's life is full of agony, anxiety, fear, and grief, complaints, sighs, suspicions, and cares, (heigh-ho, my heart is woe) full of silence and irksome solitariness!*
> *Frequenting shady bowers in discontent,*
> *To the air his fruitless clamours he will vent.*

Against the couplet, Keats annotates, 'Whose shadows the forsaken Batchelor loves Being lass-lorn.' Isabella and Lorenzo seem well on the way to Burton's more extreme state:

> the prognostication is, they will either run mad, or die. '*For if this passion continue,*' saith Aelian Montaltus, '*it makes the blood hot, thick, and black; and if the inflammation get into the brain, with continual meditation and waking, it so dries it up, that madness follows, or else they make away themselves . . . it will speedily work these effects, if it be not presently helped; They will pine away, run mad, and die upon a sudden;*' if good order be not taken . . . Go to Bedlam for examples. (pp. 347–8)

When at last Lorenzo manages to 'speak [his] grief' their woes are alleviated and they enjoy a brief period of lighthearted happiness (VIII to XI), just as Burton had prescribed as the ideal cure for love-melancholy. However, the love must remain surreptitious and hidden from Isabella's brothers. Like the brothers in Webster's *The Duchess of Malfi*, another tale of love transgressing social class, they would prefer her to marry into moneyed aristocracy rather than wed a servant. Keats had quite likely read the play,[26] as it was included in Charles Lamb's *Specimens of English Dramatic Poets, Who Lived About the Time of Shakespeare* (London: 1808), a volume which Keats owned and annotated. In tone if not narrative consistency, there is a similarity in the gruesome discovery, as Ferdinand warns his brother,

> Bosola. The office of justice is perverted quite,
> When one thief hangs another. Who shall dare
> To reveal this?
> Ferdinand.   O, I'll tell thee;
> The wolf shall find her grave, and scrape it up,
> Not to devour the corpse, but to discover
> The horrid murder.

(4.2)

Alternatively, Webster may have borrowed from Boccaccio, which is just as likely. In another intertextual twist, one of the brothers in *The Duchess* becomes mad with lycanthropia, a condition which Burton considers at length in the context of jealousy.

Far worse is to come in the second form of melancholy, after Lorenzo disappears and when Isabella learns he has been murdered. Isabella's unalleviated grief was acknowledged in the early modern world to be among the most dangerous emotional illnesses, at worst leading to the kind of passive suicide which is the poem's destined psychic territory. While 'Isabella' looks back to early modern medical lore, it also points forward once again to Freud's distinction in 'Mourning and Melancholia',[27] between on the one hand acute grief as a 'natural' mourning process which will pass, and on the other chronically debilitating melancholia. Although seen as separate conditions, the two are linked on a spectrum, since if mourning is not resolved then it can turn into the fatal melancholia. Freud sees the former as loss of the other, the latter as loss of the self. Keats's depiction consolidates the latter condition when the love-object is lost.

Keats had a personal, emotional investment in both love-melancholy and grief-induced melancholia. In May 1818 he envisaged studying 'physic, or rather Medicine again', and is 'glad at not having given away [his] Medical books'. He proceeds, 'axioms in philosophy are not axioms until they are proved upon the pulses'.[28] The phrase 'on the pulses', or '*dans le pouls*' in French textbooks, like 'proving', was a term of art in medical treatises at the time. Writing the poems was sometimes a form of self-therapy, and 'Isabella; or, The Pot of Basil' is Keats's most sombre observation of loss leading to mourning and melancholia, observed as illnesses. From the very beginning of the tale, both Isabella and Lorenzo suffer love as 'some malady' (stanza I), and as both Aileen Ward and Jack Stillinger among others have pointed out, images of disease and medicine occur throughout the poem, perhaps more frequently than in any other written by Keats.[29] Isabella 'loses' Lorenzo at three different times and in different senses. First, she thinks he has not returned from a journey, which provokes in her a sense of abandonment. Then she discovers he has been murdered, which provides the horror of realising he will not return. Finally, the pot of basil in which she has hidden his severed head is stolen by her brothers, which proves to be the fatal loss which seals her tragic fate. The sequence shows Isabella's steady deterioration into a state of profound melancholia caused by the losses, leading to her death.

Charles Lamb found 'Isabella' 'the finest thing in the volume',[30] but there have been few later critics to agree. Keats himself had reservations about the poem. These were admittedly expressed over a year after its composition, the period covering his extraordinarily rapid poetic development during 1819, suggesting that his second thoughts were a product of healthy self-criticism since he had obviously 'moved on'. By the time he came to select poems for his volume, he regarded it as 'mawkish', 'weak-sided' and 'smokeable':

> I will give you a few reasons why I shall persist in not publishing The Pot of Basil – It is too smokeable – I can get it smoak'd at the Carpenters shaving chimney much more cheaply – There is too much inexperience of live [sic], and simplicity of knowledge in it – which might do very well after one's death – but not while one is alive. There are very few would look to the reality. I intend to use more finesse with the Public. It is possible to write fine things which cannot be laugh'd at in any way. Isabella is what I should call were I a reviewer 'A weak-sided Poem' with an amusing sober-sadness about it . . .[31]

His initial preference to omit *Isabella* from the 1820 volume was reversed under persuasion by Reynolds and Woodhouse. The word 'smokeable' is usually taken to mean 'able to be ridiculed', whose origin, I suggest, may be Shakespeare's 'mockable' in *As You Like It*: 'Those that are good manners at the court are as ridiculous in the country as the behaviour of the country is most mockable at the court' (3.2.43–5). In regard to *Isabella*, he may be at least partly anxious about the dangers of 'mockable' self-revelation in choosing to present to the public his depiction of such an extreme and bizarre emotional state, involving objects that could be seen as bordering on the risible – a herb-pot and a mouldy head – a trope which a modern critic has described as 'the weirdly grotesque, laboured cultivation of a pot plant'.[32] Keats's comments suggest that it is the author more than the work which he fears is likely to be laid open to ridicule:[33] 'There is too much inexperience of live, and simplicity of knowledge in it – . . . It is possible to write fine things which cannot be laugh'd at in any way'. It lacks the distancing irony and switching perspectives of Lamia. Keats goes on to say that in his 'dramatic capacity' he enters 'fully into the feeling' of the poem's 'amusing sober-sadness', but 'in Propria Persona' he is inclined to 'quiz' it as unsympathetic critics would. Christopher Ricks frames the issue in this way: 'The word "mawkish" is usually the sign both that [Keats] is near to things that are urgent for him because his truest imaginings are involved and also that he knows how necessarily open to ridicule is his refusal to ridicule'.[34] Surely many writers are sometimes reticent in not wishing to reveal some personal connection between their fictions and their our own lives, if they appear to be drawing upon disturbing and personal psychological and emotional material in their writing. T.S. Eliot's famous assessment of *Hamlet* as a flawed work rests on exactly this doubt, since he regarded the play as faulty because Shakespeare failed to find an 'objective correlative'. Eliot surmises that the play is dealing with feelings that are 'a study to pathologists' without finding an artistic equivalent in order to distance and objectify his attempt 'to express the inexpressibly horrible'.[35] This may lead us closer to the 'reality' Keats hints at but does not fully reveal. Although the story is Boccaccio's, the menacing atmosphere is Keats's. Diane Hoeveler, for example, suggests that 'Keats never again allowed himself to be drawn into material that would expose as much of his own personal biography, veiled however darkly by the trappings of medieval or historically distanced "Romance"'. She reads 'Isabella' as 'Keats's attempt to bury his grief for his parents' deaths, repudiate his middle-class origins, and deny his attraction to "Romance", the popular Gothic ballad tradition of his day'.[36] This may be too literal in its biographical specificity (there were others in his life whom he mourned, apart from his parents, and other causes for his states of mind), but its assumptions concerning the poet's reticence about indirect, painful self-revelation do seem suggestively intrinsic to 'Isabella'.

The apparent digression concerning the 'pride and avarice' of Isabella's brothers (stanzas XIV–XVIII) according to Burton reveals another specific category of melancholy: 'Covetous men, amongst others, are most mad; they have all the symptoms of melancholy – fear, sadness, suspicion, &c. . .'[37] He gives 'Covetousness as a cause' as the heading for a chapter in which he describes a 'disease of the soul', which would explain why the brothers in both Boccaccio and Keats are later punished with guilty consciences. Burton explains, even using the metaphor of digging up a herb by the roots:

> The desire of money is the root of all evil, and they that lust after it, pierce themselves through with many sorrows, 1 Tim. vi. 10. Hippocrates therefore in his Epistle to Crateva, an herbalist, gives him this good counsel, that if it were possible, 'amongst other herbs, he should cut up that weed of covetousness by the roots, that there be no remainder left, and then know this for a certainty, that together with their bodies, thou mayst quickly cure

all the diseases of their minds. For it is indeed the pattern, image, epitome of all melancholy, the fountain of many miseries, much discontented care and woe; this 'inordinate, or immoderate desire of gain, to get or keep money,' as Bonaventure defines it: or, as Austin describes it, a madness of the soul, Gregory a torture . . . vexation of spirit, another hell.

(Book I, Section II, Member III, 12)

This is followed by a passage which in some ways anticipates, or may have influenced, Keats's detailed description of the brothers:

What makes them go into the bowels of the earth, an hundred fathom deep, endangering their dearest lives, enduring damps and filthy smells, when they have enough already, if they could be content, and no such cause to labour, but an extraordinary delight they take in riches.

Unlike Burton's covetous characters, Isabella's brothers do not risk their own lives but, transplanted into a later world of wealthy slave-owners, they delegate the miserable and dangerous pursuits to others, and their profit-obsessed mercantilism is sustained by exploitation and animal cruelty:

For them the Ceylon diver held his breath,
And went all naked to the hungry shark;
For them his ears gush'd blood; for them in death
The seal on the cold ice with piteous bark
Lay full of darts . . .

(stanza XV)

Their equally outrageous possessiveness over Isabella is also an indication of covetous melancholy, and it leads them to murder Lorenzo without compunction. In short, this section of the poem could be seen as well within Burton's taxonomy of melancholy, though very different from Isabella's state. However, the passages in the poem are so powerfully contemporary that they have stimulated overall readings of the poem as a study in affective capitalism, appealing to modern social and political viewpoints.[38] Nicholas Roe offers a literary variation on the theme, suggesting that 'An obvious "reality" [the word used by Keats in his 'smokeable' quotation], would be to recognise how the brothers' greedy, bourgeois principles are destructive of romance'.[39] Along similar lines, Jack Stillinger, emphasising the grotesque elements in the poem, suggests it is an example of Keats exploring the links between romance and anti-romance, by juxtaposing the source's 'simple plaining of a minstrel's song' with a 'tough-minded "modern" recasting'. Such a change was anticipated in the earlier sonnet, 'On Sitting Down to Read King Lear Once Again', and reappeared later in 'The Eve of St. Agnes'.[40]

The critic Evan Radcliffe describes one level of 'Isabella' as lying in 'a typical story of love and money. Its symbolic villain seems clearly to be materialism . . .', while more generally we find also 'a contrast between spiritual and material objects – or, in Keatsian terminology, between ethereal and material objects'.[41] Like Fraistat, these critics analyse 'Isabella' in terms of enacting Keats's retreat from the 'enchantment' of romance.[42] However, it is not the enchantment of love but the consequences of murder and the loss of the lover which lead to the mourning and melancholia etched in Isabella's later emotional state, and which are the central preoccupation of the poem. From the first there is little 'romance' even in the love affair.

At first told a lie by her brothers that Lorenzo has abruptly emigrated, Isabella falls into an initially 'normal' pattern of grief in response to her lover's apparent abandonment:

> She weeps alone for pleasures not to be;
> Surely she wept until the night came on.
> And then, instead of love, O misery!
> She brooded o'er the luxury alone:
>
> (stanza XXX)

'Selfishness, Love's cousin' gives way to impatient, 'feverish unrest' and then 'passion not to be subdued, | And sorrow for her love in travels rude' (stanza XXXI). Over the period from autumn to winter a slow decline in health sets in: 'So sweet Isabel by gradual decay from beauty fell, | Because Lorenzo came not' (stanzas XXXII). The brothers too are in transition under the pressure of conscience – 'Their crimes came on them' – and they become alarmed at the state of their sister 'in her snowy shroud' presaging death.

Stanzas XXXIV to XLI mark the dramatic turning point into something even more alarming, which in Freud's analysis would be explained as a transition from acute mourning for the loss of another to chronic melancholia signalling a loss of the self. In a 'medicinal' reference, the moment comes upon Isabella 'like a fierce potion, drunk by chance, | Which saves a sick man from the feather'd pall | For some few gasping moments' (stanza XXXIV), and she is visited by a vision of the dead Lorenzo. His ghost still proclaims his love, in a way that arrests Isabella's mourning and shifts it to a different, more determined emotional level, as she learns the facts of the murder, and is given directions where to find the body. In an extraordinary passage Keats expresses a consciousness of being dead (stanzas XXXVIII–XXXIX) and addressing one 'distant in Humanity'. Like Hamlet's father, Lorenzo's ghost 'mourn'd "Adieu!"– dissolv'd' (stanza XLI). From this point on, Isabella's condition turns from loss of him as a known person to loss of her own alter ego, and in effect a gradual loss of herself. She realises the turning point, from a sense of loss of the lover felt as 'simply misery', to conscious recognition of evil. Taking with her an 'aged nurse' she finds and digs up the body in the forest, severing and taking the head as a literal *memento mori*, no longer a person but a symbolic totem. The change is distilled into a disturbing image as the soiled glove that she places 'in her bosom' 'freezes utterly unto the bone' her nipples. An oddly understated phrase (which Stillinger might have in mind when he speaks of 'the grim matter-of-factness of all the "wormy circumstance"'),[43] 'And Isabella did not stamp and rave' (stanza XLVIII), marks a psychic crisis and a change into an emotionally frozen state.

Isabella steadily exhibits the kind of radical sorrow which 'takes root', described by Burton in this way (I quote leaving out some distracting details of his authorities):

> An inseparable companion, 'The mother and daughter of melancholy, her epitome, symptom, and chief cause': as Hippocrates hath it, they beget one another, and tread in a ring, for sorrow is both cause and symptom of this disease. How it is a symptom shall be shown in its place. That it is a cause all the world acknowledgeth, . . . a cause of madness, a cause of many other diseases, a sole cause of this mischief, Lemnius calls it. . . . And if it take root once, it ends in despair, . . . Chrysostom describes it to be 'a cruel torture of the soul, a most inexplicable grief, poisoned worm, consuming body and soul, and gnawing the very heart, a perpetual executioner, continual night, profound darkness, a whirlwind, a tempest, an ague not appearing, heating worse than any fire, and a battle that hath no end. It crucifies worse than any tyrant; no torture, no strappado, no bodily punishment is like unto it.' 'Tis the eagle without question which the poets feigned to gnaw Prometheus' heart, and "no heaviness is like unto the heaviness of the heart," . . .
>
>   (Book I, Section II, Memb. III, Subsect. 4)

Such debilitating sorrow caused by grief affects every bodily function: '"It hinders concoction, refrigerates the heart, takes away stomach, colour, and sleep, thickens the blood"'. Burton quotes 'My soul melteth away for very heaviness' and concludes that mourning causes 'melancholy, desperation, and sometimes death itself'. It is the very picture of Isabella at the end of the poem, from a state which 'takes root' in a literal displacement of her feelings into the basil plant, right down to the 'refrigerated' heart described by Freud as 'a profoundly painful dejection, cessation of interest in the outside world':

> And she forgot the stars, the moon, and sun,
> And she forgot the blue above the trees,
> And she forgot the dells where water runs,

And she forgot the chilly autumn breeze;
She had no knowledge when the day was done,
And the new morn she saw not: but in peace
Hung over her sweet Basil evermore,
And moisten'd it with tears unto the core.

(stanza XLIII)

To 'forget' these natural processes is, especially to a poet, an act of neglecting all that makes life worth living, and Isabella withdraws eventually from the sources of life itself. She invests all her consciousness and tears in watering the plant, which in turn naturally flourishes, 'for it drew | Nurture besides, and life, from human fears' (stanza LIV). Her fate is the kind predicted by Burton:

> As soon as Euryalus departed from Senes, Lucretia, his paramour, 'never looked up, no jests could exhilarate her sad mind, no joys comfort her wounded and distressed soul, but a little after she fell sick and died.' *But this is a gentle end, a natural death, such persons commonly make away themselves.* (p. 348)

Freud's version of melancholia seems to trace precisely the condition of Isabella: 'The ego denies the loss and strives to place within its grasp a substitute object – whether real or imaginary, in fantasy or hallucination.'[44] For Isabella the 'substitute object' is the pot of basil containing the head of Lorenzo. What follows, although repeating Boccaccio's more understated story which Keats follows relatively faithfully while extending and embroidering it with Gothic touches, seems to take the reader into more psychologically disturbing territory than the fictional context requires. The act of hacking off the head and burying it in a pot in which basil is planted takes the poem, its heroine, and author, into murky depths of some unconscious sphere of the mind where psychic transference dominates, and where dark melancholia dwells in consort with approaching death:

O Melancholy, linger here awhile!
O Music, Music! Breathe despondingly!
O Echo, Echo, from some sombre isle,
Unknown, Lethean, sigh to us – O sigh!
Spirits in grief, lift up your heads, and smile;
Lift up your heads, sweet Spirits, heavily,
And make a pale light in your cypress glooms,
Tinting with silver wan your marble tombs.

(stanza LV)

The ghastly, decaying head, manuring the lush growth of the herb, has all the trappings of a poetic symbol, akin to Eliot's 'objective correlative' for a profoundly disturbed state of mind. Seen in this way, its significance is more complex than the kind of simple imagery expected in a cameo of Gothic horror, and more also than Boccaccio's pithy narrative offers.

Why is basil chosen? Apart from the source in Boccaccio, there may be other medical reasons. The works of the Greek Paulus Aegineta, a writer who was studied in medical circles from Boccaccio's time to Keats's offers an answer. The basil to which Boccaccio and Keats referred is not the common modern cooking herb but the Greek 'Ocimum Basilicum', whose effect is described by Aegineta in translation: 'Dioscorides not only recommends it for many medicinal purposes externally; . . . but the seed, he adds, when taken in a draught, is beneficial in melancholy'.[45] This is confirmed in the work referred to, *Medical Materia Medica* of Dioscorides the ancient Greek who was considered the founder of medical botany and still regarded as an authority in both Boccaccio's and Keats's times. As late as 1810 in *A Family Herbal*, Robert John Thornton (who also refers often to Dioscorides) mentions that basil 'produces good in . . . the green sickness'.[46] There are, then, shreds of evidence traditionally linking basil with treatment of melancholy and especially in young women, as both an expression of, and complement for, Isabella's distracted, 'green' emotional condition. It was not Keats's invention but Boccaccio's, but the associations would have been appreciated by Keats.

The range of effects of the depiction also finds more eerie reverberations in Freud's descriptions of melancholia, no matter how 'deeply ambiguous and opaque' (Radden's words), specialised, and private is Freud's terminology in his essay. Many of his memorable formulations seem to apply to the final picture of Isabella as she declines to death. In her implicit and ongoing, cold hatred of her brothers, she manifests another of Freud's insights: 'the reactions expressed in [her] behavior still proceed from a mental constellation of revolt, which has then, by a certain process passed over into the crushed state of melancholia' (Freud, 248). Furthermore, the shattering of the 'object-relationship' on the death of the loved one has 'established an *identification* of the ego with the abandoned object. Thus the shadow of the object fell upon the ego . . . In this way an object-loss was transformed into an ego-loss' and the ego is 'altered by identification' (Freud, 249). Lorenzo has been transformed into mulch for a plant, and Isabella now identifies her existence wholly and obsessively with this object, doubly significant as death and life in the simultaneous horror and lush fertility of the plant, and in the lost lover it represents for her, which she strives to nurture as a still-living thing.

Isabella's loss is compounded when the brothers steal the basil-pot, dig up its contents, and confront their own guilt in the remains. On the discovery, they flee from Florence. She has now lost not only her loved one, but also the object identified with all her love, in short, herself. Again using Freud's terms, 'narcissistic identification with the object then becomes a substitute for the erotic cathexis', a term defined as morbid concentration of mental energy on one particular person, idea, or object' (p. 249), and the result is a profound 'conflict due to ambivalence' (p. 256). How can this not be so, when love is obsessively intertwined with a clod of repellent ugliness ('The thing was vile with green and livid spot' [stanza LX])? If Freud stands at the end of a long tradition stretching back to early conceptions of melancholy and debilitating 'sadness',[47] 'Isabella' can be interpreted as both a recollection of past understandings of melancholy such as Burton's, and an anticipation or premonition of Freud's future formulation, in its depiction of extreme melancholia:

> And so she pined, and so she died forlorn,
> Imploring for her Basil to the last.
> No heart was there in Florence but did mourn
> In pity of her love, so overcast.

(LXIII)

Julia Kristeva has memorably written, 'Melancholy is amorous passion's sombre lining', and it is this psychic fate to which Isabella is confined.[48]

'Isabella' came in the tailwind of *Endymion* which Keats was revising in March 1818. *Endymion* had begun with the lines, 'A thing of beauty is a joy for ever | Its loveliness increases; it will never | Pass into nothingness' (I. 1–2). But Keats by now is withdrawing from his labours over *Endymion*, and also recognising its shortcomings, which were so cruelly exploited by Tory reviewers. He could possibly see something alarming in the process of expressing dark emotions through poetry, and acknowledging that, however beautiful the surface of words, they may not be 'a joy forever'. The verse letter to Reynolds ('Dear Reynolds'), sent at exactly the same time as he was writing 'Isabella', shows a similar realisation in its description of a shift from happiness to 'horrid moods' prompted by a glimpse of predatory struggle beneath the placid beauty of the sea's surface:

>   . . . but I saw
> Too far into the sea; where every maw
> The greater on the less feeds evermore:–
> But I saw too distinct into the core
> Of an eternal fierce destruction . . .[49]

Something analogous to the 'horrid moods, | Moods of one's mind' in the verse letter could be said of the discrepancy between the appearance of Isabella's flourishing basil plant and its dark psychological and physiological referent, watered by her tears, 'Whence thick, and green, and beautiful it grew, | So that it smelt more balmy than its peers | Of Basil-tufts in Florence' (LIV). There is also an analogy to be drawn with the lyrical surface of the poem and its murky subject matter. The poem is explicit that the buried head has its roots in a dismaying place of 'human fears':

> for it drew
> Nurture besides, and life, from human fears,
> From the fast mouldering head there shut from view:
> So that the jewel, safely casketed,
> Came forth, and in perfumed leaflets spread.
>
> (LIV)

It is not difficult to see the basil plant as holding the ambiguous status of the poem itself, as 'a thing of beauty' whose genesis lies in material which includes the body of a murdered man and inconsolable and suicidal melancholy. These, in turn, have come not only from Keats's literary source but also his own imagination, as a poet who has spent much of his own life in contemplation of melancholy, and is engaged in turning it into poetry.[50] Even the transfixed description of the dead body with its weirdly described 'Pale limbs at bottom of a crystal well' and the 'fast mouldering head' – 'The thing was vile and green with livid spot' ... 'and past his loamed ears | Had made a miry channel for his tears' – may be yet another momentary flashback to anatomy classes at Guy's, presided over by a sympathetic but unflinching Astley Cooper carving up decomposing corpses stolen from graves by 'resurrection men' to service the medical profession. Even out of such recollected horrors can come poetry, and works of enduring aesthetic quality such as 'Lycidas' and *In Memoriam* often spring from suffering, loss and emotional trauma. The beauty of a poem is rooted in the all-too-mortal melancholia of the poet, and is at least metaphorically watered by his own tears. A variation on this formulation of poetic self-reflexivity is given by Tilottama Rajan, who argues that art is born from neurosis, although this risks underplaying the degree of artistic control and self-reflective knowledge we find constantly in Keats's poems.[51] As elsewhere in his works, the healer and the patient are one. At the very end of 'Isabella', after her death, Keats is licensed by Boccaccio's conclusion – 'an excellent ditty was composed thereof, beginning thus: "Cruell and unkinde was the Christian, That robd me of my Basiles blisse &c."'[52] – focus attention on the poem *as poem* rather than any longer as a state of mind within a fiction:

And a sad ditty of this story born
From mouth to mouth through all the country pass'd:
Still is the burthen sung – "O cruelty,
"To steal my Basil-pot away from me!"

(LXIII)

This reference to the story-as-story reprises the earlier authorial request
for a 'pardon' from the original creator:

O eloquent and famed Boccaccio!
Of thee we now should ask forgiving boon,
And of thy spicy myrtles as they blow,
And of thy roses amorous of the moon,
And of thy lilies, that do paler grow
Now they can no more hear thy ghittern's tune,
For venturing syllables that ill beseem
The quiet glooms of such a piteous theme.

(stanza XIX)

Now that Boccaccio has gone the way of Lorenzo and the ghittern is
mute, all that remains of that writer are the myrtles, roses, lilies which
are his poems (if that is the force of Keats's 'thy'), as well as the poetic
imitation of a deferential later poet, recreating 'The quiet glooms of such
a piteous theme' in his tale of melancholy. At least the tale recounting
loss is not itself lost, and can be recreated:

Fair reader, at the old tale take a glance,
For here, in truth, it doth not well belong
To speak: – O turn thee to the very tale,
And taste the music of that vision pale.

Through the process of adaptation, something lost may have been refound,
but in such a different form that the contrast elegiacally accentuates the
loss of a 'pale vision' from the past, representing the historical time in
which Boccaccio had written his 'old tale'. The fact that Boccaccio himself
builds into his tale a sense that the events occurred long ago in the past,
were preserved by word of mouth in a ballad and then recounted in his
own poem, is another, subtle reminder of art as the result of some distant,
loss being continually rediscovered and re-experienced through poetry.
Later poems in the 1820 collection will explicitly return to this refrain.

'The Eve of St Agnes'

The ritual enacted in 'The Eve of St Agnes' was suggestively mentioned
in *The Anatomy of Melancholy* on a page side-marked and underlined

by Keats. Burton, in describing the symptoms of young love, mentions lovers' compulsion to versify their feelings:

> But above all the other symptoms of lovers, this is not lightly to be over-passed, that likely of what condition soever, if once they be in love, they turn to their ability, rhymers, ballad makers, and poets.

Examples follow, among them one allusion, veiled by a misprint, so brief that it could be missed in the blink of an eye:

> *They will in all places be doing thus, young folks especially, reading love stories, talking of this or that young man, such a fair maid, singing, telling or hearing lascivious tales, scurrilous tunes, such objects are their sole delight, their continual meditation, . . . an earnest longing comes hence, pruriens corpus, pruriens anima, amorous conceits, tickling thoughts, sweet and pleasant hopes; hence it is, they can think, discourse willingly, or speak almost of no other subject. 'Tis their only desire, if it may be done by art, to see their husband's picture in a glass, they'll give anything to know when they shall be married, how many husbands they shall have, by cromnyomantia, a kind of divination with onions laid on the altar on Christmas eve, or by fasting on St. Anne's [sic] eve or night, to know who shall be their first husband . . . This love is the cause of all good conceits, neatness, exornations, plays, elegancies, delights, pleasant expressions, sweet motions, and gestures, joys, comforts, exultancies, and all the sweetness of our life.*

> (p. 341, Keats's side-lining and underlining)

It is a curiously carnal myth to find associated with a serially assaulted early martyr who proclaimed Christ was her only lover, was burned at the stake and finally beheaded at the age of twelve or thirteen, and canonised as patron saint of chastity, virgins and rape victims. Her feast day is 21 January so the 'Eve' falls on 20 January. The superstition, 'by fasting on St. Anne's eve or night, to know who shall be their first husband . . .' was a brief stimulus, if not full-blown source, for 'The Eve of St Agnes', and Burton directly links the superstition to poetic creation.

According to Woodhouse, it was also suggested to Keats as a subject for a poem by Isabella Jones on Sunday 17 January 1819. He began composing on the following day, two days before the Eve, completing it on 2 February and revising in September. It was written in Bedhampton, when Keats was staying with the Snooks in their mill-house at Bedhampton, and a guest house in Chichester (both spots now marked by blue plaques). The setting, with its detailed descriptions, is generally assumed to be based on Stansted Park House between Chichester and Bedhampton, which Keats visited in the company of Charles Brown and the Snooks. They attended the consecration of the adjoining, neomedieval chapel on 25 January,[53] and although reluctant and critical of the religious trappings and service, Keats was to allow the architecture to feed richly into 'The Eve', as Robert Gittings recounts in unforgettable detail.[54] Apart from the reference to 'St. Anne's eve' and perhaps the general aloofness of the narrative voice observing *'young folks especially, reading love stories'*, the poem owes less to Burton than do the shifting styles in 'Lamia' and the psychological subject matter of 'Isabella'. Unlike the two previous poems in *1820*, it has no sustained source, but in conception and narrative direction is influenced primarily by the love and elopement story in *Romeo and Juliet* (complete with nurse), and in style, setting and atmosphere (what Keats refers to as 'the colouring of St. Agnes's eve'),[55] to the more recent genres, Gothic romance and, to a lesser extent, graveyard poetry. Ann Radcliffe's Gothic tales especially hover insistently, and Keats's facetious comment on his 'fine mother Radcliff names' refers aptly to 'The Eve of St. Agnes' in more than just name.[56] In the Keatsian 'anatomy of melancholy' with which I am framing *1820*, he is now moving forward in time from the Burtonian inspiration to the literary and cultural forms of melancholy in the Renaissance and eighteenth century.

One book in particular may have been in Keats's imagination in his 'colouring' of this poem and the next, Radcliffe's Gothic novel *The Mysteries of Udolpho* (1794). It was certainly read by Keats, and I suggest this work contributed especially to the air of radical ambiguity that hangs over Porphyro's actions and motives. He has been variously interpreted by critics as anything from a benign and entitled suitor to a malevolent intruder and even rapist.[57] Intruder he may be, but unknown to Madeline he is not, since Angela addresses him by name ('"Mercy, Porphyro! Hie thee from this place"' [stanza XI]) and so does Madeline herself (XXXV). However, grounds for the more sinister possibility may have crept in from the influence of one climactic scene in Volume 2, Chapter VI of *Udolpho*, where there are two intruders. Both are villainous but the narrative sequence is strikingly similar. Emily, the heroine, is stalked in her bedroom by would-be suitor Count Morano. Unlike Madeline, she retires to bed fully clothed with a sense of 'prophetic apprehension'. She sinks into a 'disturbed slumber' (Keats writes, 'slumberous tenderness') and 'as sometimes occur in dreams' noises awaken her, sounding like 'the undrawing of rusty bolts' (compare Keats's 'The key turns, and the door upon its hinges groans'). The lamp 'spread so feeble a light through the apartment, that the remote parts of it were lost in shadow' (Keats: 'A chain-droop'd lamp was flickering by each door'). A 'mysterious form' 'seemed to glide along' (Keats: 'They glide along, like phantoms, into the wide hall; | Like phantoms, to the iron porch, they glide'). The verbal likenesses may be too close to Gothic conventions to claim *Udolpho* as a clear source for 'St Agnes', but the way both Radcliffe and Keats create effects of material objects seeming to have an inner life of their own while people become wraith-like suggests the common generic inheritance of the Gothic novel, with its insistent emphasis on a prevailing atmosphere mingling melancholy and menace. The intruder, Count Morano, beseeches Emily 'to fear nothing' and ardently professes his love for her. Revealing the villainy of the castle's owner, Montoni, he suggests,

Can I love you, and abandon you to his power? Fly, then, fly from this gloomy prison, with a lover, who adores you! I have bribed a servant of the castle to open the gates, and, before tomorrow's dawn, you shall be far on the way to Venice.

(Compare Keats's '"Arise – arise! ... Let us away ... Arise! arise! my love, and fearless be"' [XXXIX]). Understandably terrified, Emily realises that her only hope of escaping the castle is to 'submit herself to the protection of this man', who she is now aware is more evil than he had appeared. He continues to urge her: '"Let us go, then," said Morano, eagerly kissing her hand, and rising, "my carriage waits, below the castle walls." She resists, and the scene erupts into violence when a voyeuristic second man, Montoni himself, enters and wounds Morano. Although the moral curve involving two evil men and the conclusion are very different from Keats's poem, it does seem from the similarities in presentation and echoes of language that he is building upon some details in Radcliffe's suspenseful presentation. In doing so he may, possibly inadvertently, have imported the presentation of Morano's moral ambiguity, which becomes attached to Porphyro through the plot similarity and some imagery. The problematical elements, then, may be attributed to the genre itself of Gothic melodrama, since few men in Radcliffe are wholly trustworthy and virtuous, and all are regarded as at least potential villains. The kind of melancholy depicted in the novel is built upon the natural fears and night terrors of a vulnerable woman entrapped in a gloomy, Gothic setting, threatened by hostile figures around her.

At a more conscious level, however, Keats seems to be appealing more to the memory of *Romeo and Juliet*, in which elopement is a consensual act which frees the woman through love from her constricting family environment, rather than to the inbuilt Gothic air of menace which provides the surrounding atmosphere. As Shakespeare's lovers intuit, in a play where the word 'fear' occurs twenty-five times, even without doubting each other's virtue, the situation is intrinsically fraught with doubts and is scary enough, since the unlived future requires a recklessly impetuous decision. The ending of 'St Agnes', whether considered 'happy' or otherwise, enacts a liberation of the poem itself, this time from the present tense, moral relativities and 'gloomy prison' of present, claustrophobic dread and melancholy, into a more bracing but potentially more realistic, albeit stormy existence: 'And they are gone, ay ages long ago | These lovers fled away into the storm'. Something is lost – Madeline's innocence at least, since the rose cannot shut 'and be a bud again', but more is gained by escaping into the future by confronting the world beyond dreams and romance.

However we evaluate the 'ardour of the pursuer'[58] of Porphyro as moral agent, we should not minimise Madeline's emotions, which provide the poem's primary affective register, a prevailing sense of solitary melancholy. The 'ardent revelry' of the feast 'With plume, tiara, and all rich array' and the spirit of 'old Romance' give way, as the narrator 'sole-thoughted' turns to 'one Lady there, | Whose soul had brooded, all that wintry day | On love, and winged saint Agnes' saintly care . . .', whose legend she has learned from 'old dames'. 'Upon the honeyed middle of the night' she retires 'supperless', observing all the 'ceremonies' and hoping to see her dream-lover. She does not hear 'The music, yearning like a God in pain', and she dances 'with vague, regardless eyes', breathing quickly in anticipation. If not already in love, she is ready for love, distracted and apprehensive of what she expects to be a revealing, nocturnal dream: 'her heart was voluble, | Paining with eloquence her balmy side', like a 'tongueless nightingale', an image reminding of Ovid's raped Philomel who turned into a nightingale. She falls first into a 'wakeful swoon' and then is by 'the poppied warmth of sleep oppressed', 'blissfully havened both from joy and pain'. Her awakening to Porphyro's lute music comes as 'a painful change', and she begins to weep at the difference between his dream-presence and the 'pallid, chill, and drear' reality: 'No dream, alas! alas! And woe is mine'. She is torn between pleading with the man not to abandon her and feeling the vulnerability of 'a poor deceived thing – | A dove forlorn and sick with unpruned wing'. Just as critics are divided over Porphyro, so are they on Madeline's feelings, between those who emphasise her fear, seeing it as a 'hoodwinking' (hooding a bird to train it into obedience) in a state of unwilling, 'stuperous insensibility' (Stillinger's phrase),[59] and those who gravitate to the implicit hope of lovers embodied in the romance of St Agnes Eve. Susan Wolfson has stressed the passive side of Madeline as 'innocent dreamer, and object of rapt devotion',[60] while Mary Arseneau sees her more in terms of the ambiguous feelings she generates in Porphyro (and perhaps Keats) as 'saintly and enchanting' but also a 'locus of female agency and as a potential threat to Porphyro'.[61] However, the fact that her main desire is not to be abandoned by Porphyro and left to live in the inhospitable family home, but to elope with him, suggests that hope finally quashes fear. It does seem possible to keep both readings in suspension, seeing Madeline's emotions as rapidly and plausibly progressing through feelings of entrapment, enchantment, hopeful dreaming, waking confusion, a sense of betrayal, dread, fear, and finally resolution. In a curiously prophetic way her responses mirror Elisabeth Kübler-Ross's 'five stages of grief' – denial, anger, bargaining, depression, acceptance[62] – acknowledging that young love can include grief at the loss of one life in hazardous pursuit of another. In Burton's multiple, often conflicting, observations on lovers' feelings and behaviour, all such states are symptomatic of volatile, changeable love-melancholy, which by its nature mingles joy and anxiety. In the imaginative worlds of both Burton and Keats, love is a many-splendoured melancholy, subjecting its victims to tumultuous emotions they have never experienced before, and never will again.

Though there is no churchyard in 'The Eve of St. Agnes', the genre of graveyard poetry leaves its traces at the beginning and end, in the figures of the Beadsman and Angela. The former is defined in terms of religion since his task as an almsman is to say prayers for the dead:

> Numb were the Beadsman's fingers, while he told
> His rosary, and while his frosted breath,
> Like pious incense from a censer old,
> Seem'd taking flight for heaven, without a death,
> Past the sweet Virgin's picture, while his prayer he saith.
>
> (stanza I)

After 'this patient, holy man' says his prayers, he takes his lamp and barefooted moves 'Along the chapel aisle by slow degrees: | The sculptur'd dead, on each side, seem to freeze' (stanza II). It is a kind of indoor graveyard, no doubt inspired by the interior of the Stansted chapel. The third stanza indicates that he himself is destined to die this very night – 'already had his deathbed run' – but he resolves to stay awake all night and do his duty, 'for sinners' sakes to grieve'. The kind of melancholy engendered in graveyard poetry, as distinct from the less soothing Gothic melancholy, is contemplation of the dead and the transience of the mortal condition within a religious context,[63] and the Beadsman is a vehicle for such sentiments.

Angela similarly defines herself when she pleads with Porphyro not to carry out his plan:

> "Ah, why wilt thou affright a feeble soul?
> A poor, weak, palsy-stricken churchyard thing,
> Whose passing-bell may ere the midnight toll;

Whose prayers for thee, each morn and evening,
Were never missed . . ."

(stanza XVIII)

By the end of the poem the prophecies of death are fulfilled for these
elderly characters, both described as 'meagre':

Angela the old
Died palsy-twitched, with meagre face deform;
The Beadsman, after thousand aves told,
For aye unsought for slept among his ashes cold.

(stanza XLII)

Woodhouse wrote that Keats wished 'to leave on the reader a sense of
pettish disgust, bringing Old Angela in (only) dead stiff & ugly. – He says
he likes that the poem should leave off with this Change of Sentiment
. . .'.[64] Although here he was commenting on a harsher, revised draft,
the 'Change of Sentiment' still operates. What has been a poem set
in Gothic gloom, foregrounding narrative suspense, entrapped youth,
briefly fulfilled love, and promise of escape and a fresh start, is given
a closure which includes a pensive, death-laden spirit closer to Gray's
Elegy in a Country Churchyard, reinforcing the impression of a bleaker
reality existing on the edge of the poem's boundaries.

However, such a sombre note applies only to the world left behind by
Porphyro and Madeline, if their flight is seen as a positive and healthy
rite of passage away from the environment marked first by drunken
violence and then death of ancients. This may inadvertently explain why
Keats did not include 'La Belle Dame Sans Merci' in the collection. If he
had so chosen, then it may well have followed 'The Eve of St. Agnes',
since a song of this title is sung by Porphyro in the 'Eve' itself:

Awakening up, he took her hollow lute,–
Tumultuous,– and, in chords that tenderest be,
He play'd an ancient ditty, long since mute,
In Provence call'd, "La belle dame sans mercy":
Close to her ear touching the melody; –

An obvious misunderstanding of inclusion would be created that Keats's
own 'La Belle Dame' is that very song. As the most Burtonian, melancholy vision of love, it would be an inappropriate interpolation in this
context, with its vision of torpid passivity and of love as paralysing
entrapment, at odds with the apparent freedom of the lovers in 'St.
Agnes' in their rite of passage. Instead, Keats follows 'St. Agnes' with
a poem dealing explicitly with the entrancing properties of music itself,
maintaining the more positive and hopeful tonal direction set by the
lovers' flight.

'Ode to a Nightingale'

What other reasons might have inclined Keats to follow 'The Eve of St Agnes' with 'Ode to a Nightingale' in the 1820 volume? No doubt various answers can be given, for example, the prompt given by the transitional reference to Madeline as the 'tongueless nightingale' (stanza XXIII), her experience of a 'waking dream' into startling reality anticipating the end of 'Nightingale', and near-repetitions of imagery such as 'Into her dream he melted, as the rose | Blendeth its odour with the violet – | Solution sweet' and 'Fast fading violets covered up in leaves; | And mid-May's eldest child, | The coming musk-rose . . .'. (It is worth noting that in Burton's *Anatomy*, references to the rose and violet come frequently in tandem.)

There may be another surprising link with Radcliffe's *The Mysteries of Udolpho*. If Madeline's situation is comparable to Emily's in the novel, we notice also insistent usages of the nightingale image, regularly associated by Radcliffe with melancholy moods:

> The sun was now set, and, recalling her thoughts from their melancholy subject, she continued her walk; for the pensive shade of twilight was pleasing to her, and the nightingales from the surrounding groves began to answer each other in the long-drawn, plaintive note, which always touched her heart; while all the fragrance of the flowery thickets, that bounded the terrace, was awakened by the cool evening air, which floated so lightly among their leaves, that they scarcely trembled as it passed.
>
> (vol. 4, ch. X)

For Keats, the bird's song is a 'plaintive anthem'. And again:

> Overcome by these recollections, she, at length, left the spot, and walked slowly into the woods, where the softened music, floating at a distance, soothed her melancholy mind. The moon threw a mellow light among the foliage; the air was balmy and cool, and Emily, lost in thought, strolled on, without observing whither, till she perceived the sounds sinking afar off, and an awful stillness round her, except that, sometimes, the nightingale beguiled the silence with 'Liquid notes, that close the eye of day'.
>
> (vol. 3, ch. XIII)

The final quotation comes from Milton's sonnet on the nightingale. In the novel, although Emily is associated with the nightingale, it is not only she who hears the 'mourning' note (vol. 1, ch. XXX) as 'pensive', but also her lover who, like Porphyro, prepares a delicious meal:

> He loved the soothing hour, when the last tints of light die away; when the stars, one by one, tremble through aether, and are reflected on the dark

mirror of the waters; that hour, which, of all others, inspires the mind with pensive tenderness, and often elevates it to sublime contemplation. When the moon shed her soft rays among the foliage, he still lingered, and his pastoral supper of cream and fruits was often spread beneath it. Then, on the stillness of night, came the song of the nightingale, breathing sweetness, and awakening melancholy.

(vol. 1, ch. 1)

Radcliffe proceeds to compose her own poem linking the nightingale, music, and melancholy:

> To music's softest sounds they dance away the hour,
> Till moon-light steals down among the trembling leaves,
> And checquers all the ground, and guides them to the bow'r,
> The long haunted bow'r, where the nightingale grieves.
> Then no more they dance, till her sad song is done,
> But, silent as the night, to her mourning attend;
> And often as her dying notes their pity have won,
> They vow all her sacred haunts from mortals to defend.

Of course, and for obvious reasons, the mellifluous song of the elusive nightingale has always been a common and symbolic trope for poets, and Burton in the *Anatomy* had linked it with melancholy in his metaphor for the 'modest man, one that hath grace, a generous spirit' who, 'as a nightingale, ... dies for shame if another bird sing better, he languisheth and pineth away in the anguish of his spirit' (Book I, Memb. III, Subsect VI). But the specific connections drawn in *The Mysteries of Udolpho*, a book close to Keats's memory when he wrote these poems, seem too close to ignore. The ode is also peppered with favourite 'mother Radcliffe' vocabulary and images used in *Udolpho*, such as 'glooms', 'dewy', verdure', 'plaintive', 'viewless', 'haunt' and 'forlorn' ('His forlorn and melancholy look', ch. 5, and the word is repeated seventeen more times). The literal 'Silent as the night' is touched into metaphor in Keats's 'tender is the night'. Radcliffe's line, 'whose pathless sod is darkly seen' which links 'sod' and (almost) 'darkling', comes in her interpolated poem, 'To Melancholy', sung with 'gentle sadness' by the heroine to the tune of her lute (vol. 4, ch. XVIII). Grammatically, her poem asks the 'lonely spirit' of the song repeatedly to 'Guide me ...' and 'Lead, ...' through an imagined, moonlit forest. Once again, there is not enough to claim Radcliffe's novel as a major source, but enough to compare the emotional landscape, as well as a shared vocabulary of melancholy. Such echoes from *Udolpho* take their place among a host of semi-buried literary allusions in the 'Ode' – to Horace, Marlowe, Spenser, Drayton, Milton, Dryden, Shirley, Burton,[65] Charlotte Smith, Wordsworth, Shakespeare,[66] and Coleridge who in turn quotes from

Milton and points out that the collocation of nightingale and melancholy is not inevitable but a projection of a poet's mind:

> And hark! The Nightingale begins its song,
> 'Most musical, most melancholy' bird!
> A melancholy bird? Oh! Idle thought!
> In Nature there is nothing melancholy,
> But some night-wandering man whose heart was pierced
> With the remembrance of a grievous wrong,
> Or slow distemper, or neglected love,
> (And so, poor wretch! Filled all things with himself,
> And made all gentle sounds tell back the tale
> Of his own sorrow) he, and such as he,
> First named these notes a melancholy strain.
> And many a poet echoes the conceit.[67]

So full of echoes from 'many a poet' is Keats's ode that its subject is as much poetry itself as the nightbird's song or music in general. The subject of nightingales was one of several discussed by Coleridge, Keats and his former demonstrator at Guy's, Joseph Henry Green, when they ambled together at Coleridge's 'alderman-after dinner pace' on a walk towards Highgate in mid-April 1819, a couple of weeks before the ode was written.[68]

It is music as representing the sense of sound which is the ode's principal subject, dominating it as surely as did eyesight in 'Lamia', and stimulating its own unique form of melancholy. Leigh Hunt detected in the poem 'that mixture in it of real melancholy and imaginative relief',[69] implying that melancholy is presented as an illness which can be given 'relief' or remedied by poetry. In our own day of mass auditory reproduction, we can listen to a musical piece over and over again to our heart's desire, even the recorded sound of a nightingale, but in Keats's time this was clearly not possible. All that could be done by way of repetition were the little 'chamber concerts' of music in which each person simulated an instrument, at coterie evenings hosted first by Cowden Clarke Senior for his students and then by Hunt and Novello in Keats's earlier days when his 'heart | Was warmed luxuriously by divine Mozart; | By Arne delighted, or by Handel madden'd'.[70] In these, the experience may have been close to achieving Duke Orsino's wish at the beginning of *Twelfth Night*, in words which surely also influenced Keats's 'Ode':

> If music be the food of love, play on;
> Give me excess of it, that, surfeiting,
> The appetite may sicken, and so die.
> That strain again! it had a dying fall:
> O, it came o'er my ear like the sweet sound,

That breathes upon a bank of violets,
Stealing and giving odour.

(1.1.1–7)

However, the rarely heard music of the nightingale could not 'play on' at the volition of the human auditor, and its self-contained and evanescent song, heard by chance, once completed is gone. The realisation intensifies the already poignant quality of music itself, a medium fleetingly enacted in time alone, rarely representing a material 'subject-matter' but referring only to its own created, imaginative and affective world. The medium epitomises the intersection of the fleeting and the eternal. Providing moments that are timeless while they last, it is yet of necessity bound by time, not existing beforehand or sustained permanently. As Coleridge noted, it is also the art form which is open for the listener to project upon it some personal and often overwhelming emotional experience. This is the kind of melancholy which Keats dwells upon in 'Ode to a Nightingale'.

In this case melancholy, in one sense or another, predominates at each stage in the ode. Significantly, it is a word that begins the sequence of thoughts, 'envy' with its implications of jealousy and desire, and a word that ends it, 'forlorn, the very word ...', its root implying 'lost'. The former lies in Burton's territory, signalled by a subtle echo. The passage is not marked by Keats but it occurs in one which he has marked, when Burton is writing gloomily on 'Cures of Jealousy':

> no remedy but patience ... There is no other cure but time to wear it out, *Injuriarum remedium est oblivio*, as if they had drunk a draught of Lethe in Trophonius' den: to conclude, age will bereave her of it, dies *dolorem minuit*, time and patience must end it.
>   The mind's affections patience will appease,
>   It passions kills, and healeth each disease.

(p. 464)

The connection is that the poet's 'heartache' is caused by a kind of empathising 'envy' for the nightingale's state, in 'being too happy in thine happiness', as it sings 'of summer in full-throated ease' in self-absorbed rapture. John A. Minahan, in *Word Like a Bell*, the book-length study of music in Keats, glosses in this way:

> The poet's heart aches, but it does so because it is 'too happy'. The poet wishes to join in essence with the bird's song, and the act of trying to do so makes him ever more aware of himself, of his own happily aching heart.[71]

The symptoms of the poet's dejected spirit, curable only by 'time and patience', are the kind that can be induced by narcotic drugs, as Burton says, '*Injuriarum remedium est oblivion* ('the remedy for the injury is oblivion'), as if one has drunk a 'draught' sending him Lethe-wards':

> My heart aches, and a drowsy numbness pains
> My sense, as though of hemlock I had drunk,
> Or emptied some dull opiate to the drains
> One minute past, and Lethe-wards had sunk.

As Gareth Evans has pointed out, hemlock was seen as an alternative to opium in pain-killing and sleep-inducing properties, and the combination of juices from the two was a powerful mix that would cause 'easeful death'.[72] Burton, speaking of euthanasia and 'Prognostics of Melancholy', had told of inhabitants of 'the island of Choa' where, 'with poppy or hemlock they prevented death' (Partition I, Sect. IV, Memb. 1), requiring eventual 'voluntary death': 'let him free himself with his own hands from this tedious life, as from a prison, or suffer himself to be freed by others'. Meanwhile, Burton's favourite, less dangerous panaceas for 'Mending the Temperament', which can at least distract if not cure the melancholic, are music, dance, and especially '*a cup of wine or strong drink*' which '*procures sleep*', recommended in a lengthy passage side-marked by Keats: ' *"it makes those which are otherwise dull, to exhale and evaporate like frankincense, or quicken" (Xenophon adds) as oil doth fire . . . And that which is all in all to my purpose, it takes away fear and sorrow*' (p. 126). Keats's speaker, taking the advice, calls for 'a draught of vintage!', 'a beaker full of the warm South':

> With beaded bubbles winking at the brim,
> And purple-stained mouth;
> That I might drink, and leave the world unseen,
> And with thee fade away into the forest dim.

However, locked in the melancholic state which can be cured only by time, the poet-speaker cannot yet 'fade far away, and quite forget' nor find 'oblivion', since he is always mindful of others sharing the melancholy consciousness of disease and mortality,

> The weariness, the fever, and the fret
> Here, where men sit and hear each other groan;
> Where palsy shakes a few, sad, last gray hairs,
> Where youth grows pale, and spectre-thin, and dies;
> Where but to think is to be full of sorrow
> And leaden-eyed despairs,
> Where Beauty cannot keep her lustrous eyes,
> Or new Love pine at them beyond to-morrow.

A succession of critics over the years have noted that Keats is here reliving memories of the incurable, terminally ill patients he attended at Guy's Hospital, of helplessly watching his mother and brother die of wasting disease, and asking the nagging and unanswerable question about the arbitrariness of disease, why 'Women have cancers'.[73] Perversely, the imagined rapture of the nightingale's song has only accentuated the bedrock mood of melancholy in the poet, who is perhaps drunk by this stage, explaining the 'dull brain' which 'perplexes and retards', or at the least succumbing to the cocktail of narcotics which will lift inhibitions that burden his imagination.

Wine, the elixir of Bacchus, having failed to lift his spirits, the poet through an act of willed agency ('Away! Away! for I will fly to thee') finds his spirits roused 'on the viewless wings of Poesy'. The act of surrendering to the affective medium of music engenders a state where time either 'stands still' or expands to infinity in an experience of ecstasy, a Lacanian *jouissance* of pleasure pushed to pain. As Hrileena Ghosh mentions, the 'reverie' which the poet describes constitutes an escape from self which, in contemporary medical accounts, could be a dangerous excitement which could lead to illness,[74] as Burton also had warned. Transported, the poet enters a state of mental synaesthesia where all senses become activated through the sense of sound. Since the realm of sound alone is 'viewless' ('here there is no light') the only visibility is imaginary, 'verdurous glooms and winding mossy ways'. Although the poet 'cannot see' the flowers around his feet, yet the other senses are so keenly awakened that he can 'in embalmed darkness, guess each sweet', smell summer's aromas, and hear 'The murmurous haunt of flies on summer eves'. 'Darkling I listen' is central to the poem's movement, providing its own light as in the blind Milton's 'No light, but rather darkness visible' (*Paradise Lost* 1, 63). The word 'darkling' is used by Shakespeare in *A Midsummer Night's Dream*, *Antony and Cleopatra* and *King Lear*, but the more immediate allusion is to another passage by Milton in *Paradise Lost*, also referring to the nightingale: 'As the wakeful bird sings darkling, | And in shadiest Covert hid | Tunes her nocturnal note' (III.37–40).[75] It can be used as verb (becoming dark), noun (a state of darkness), adjective or adverb (lying in darkness), and in Keats's ode the '-ing' word evokes a continuous present, suspending time in timelessness at the moment of mental surrender. A feeling of expanded consciousness created by 'such an ecstasy' of beautiful music leads to a swooning desire for Burtonian oblivion, a death-wish – 'Now more than ever seems it rich to die' – in order to avert or delay a transition back to the earth-bound reality prefigured in 'To thy high requiem become a sod'. In the extraordinarily compressed literary intertextuality

of the ode, Keats probably recalled Othello's 'If it were now to die |
'Twere now to be most happy' (2.1), and the state is also analogous to
that of a lover mentioned by Burton, whose words are side-marked by
Keats: '*He could find in his heart to be killed instantly, lest if he live
longer, some sorrow or sickness should contaminate his joys*' (p. 305).
The bird itself, the poet believes, can never die – 'thou wast not born for
death, immortal Bird!' – so long as the singular, 'unseen' bird is concep-
tualised as quintessential song itself, which will always be repeated over
the centuries if not by the same creature. The disembodied, beautiful
sound was heard as much 'in ancient days by emperor and clown', and
in the state of exiled melancholy in the 'sad heart of Ruth, when, sick for
home, | She stood in tears amid the alien corn'. It still has the capacity to
transport the listener to another realm, to 'charm' (captivate, enchant),
creating 'magic casements, opening on the foam | Of perilous seas, in
faery lands forlorn', all products of the awakened imagination, abstract-
ing the poet from a burdening sense of self. At this stage of the poem,
consistent with the subject of the essence of music as a transitory, deeply
affective art, the poet's linguistic intervention creates a dismaying transition, in the choice of a word, 'Forlorn!' which 'tolls' the poet like a bell
back from the expansive and spell-bound universality of the music to his
own 'sole self', locking him once again in time, space, and subjectivity.
The music fades as the nightingale flies into the next valley, and the poet
finds himself alone and left dazed, tricked by the 'deceiving elf' of his
own imagination, and barely able to categorise the ecstatic emotional
state evoked by music, now that it has stopped: 'Was it a vision, or a
waking dream? | Fled is that music: – Do I wake or sleep?'. Burton uses
'waking dream' twice, first in Book I and secondly in the midst of pages
on despair and guilty conscience. Keats has not marked the phrase itself
but the whole section is marked quite heavily. Burton is reflecting on
hope as an antidote to despair:

> all kinds [of despair] are opposite to hope, that sweet moderator of passions,
> as Simonides calls it; I do not mean that vain hope which fantastical fellows
> feign to themselves, which according to Aristotle is *insomnium vigilantium*, a
> waking dream; but this divine hope which proceeds from confidence, and is
> an anchor to a floating soul . . .
>
> (p. 563)

Aristotle's 'hope is a waking dream' does not occur in his own works
but was attributed to him by Diogenes Laertius in *Lives of Eminent
Philosophers* which Keats was unlikely to have read. The collocation of
'fantastical', 'feign', and 'waking dream' in Burton's sentence perhaps
gives enough reason to regard it as a prompt for Keats's desire for

hopeful wish-fulfilment, and the image of 'an anchor to a floating soul' adds a suggestive touch. The final words in the ode call into question the reality and truth status of the transporting, mood-changing experience as a whole, asking whether the dream-like suspension of time and expansion of consciousness in rapt oneness with the music, create its own reality, as a more richly sensuous, all-inclusive yet immaterial state than the desolate isolation of the 'sole self' once again left mentally stranded in time.

The kind of melancholy fuelling 'Ode to a Nightingale' seems to fall within Burton's category of those states of melancholy which can be alleviated temporarily but not permanently cured. These include the most inescapably self-conscious emotions such as jealousy and envy, which are motivated by desire of others' happiness, and which leave the sufferer in an intensely painful awareness of a 'sole self' anchored in time, place and consciousness. Such moods can be lifted by the fleeting distraction of music, moments which are insubstantial and illusory products of 'fancy', imagination, 'vision', 'dream': 'Adieu! the fancy cannot cheat so well | As she is fam'd to do, deceiving elf', in which case the melancholy is deepened rather than cured. (Some critics, such as John Jones, believe Keats's intended word was 'fain'd' ['feigned'].)[76] A remedy lies in the act of writing the poem in celebration of such instants of distraction, but when the song ends, the poem also ends where it began, and melancholy returns. Burton, in Book I of *The Anatomy of Melancholy*, quotes Erasmus who pessimistically suggests that this kind of melancholy is, sadly, a mark of mortal experience, the condition to which only 'fools' can remain oblivious:

> Erasmus vindicates fools from this melancholy catalogue, because they have most part moist brains and light hearts; they are free from ambition, envy, shame and fear; they are neither troubled in conscience, nor macerated with cares, to which our whole life is most subject.
>
> (Book I, Memb. III, Subsec. II)

'Ode on a Grecian Urn'

It is not difficult to see why 'Ode on a Grecian Urn' follows 'Ode to a Nightingale' since they are natural companions, both dealing with the relationship between art and time. The lines 'Heard melodies are sweet, but those unheard | Are sweeter' explain literally why this poem follows 'Nightingale', as attention moves from sound to silence. The twinned status of music and visual art as complementary reflections on the nature of art is indicated by the fact that both odes were initially published in the journal *Annals of Fine Art* (July 1819 and January 1820 respectively). They also both deal with kinds of melancholy that can never finally be cured but only alleviated.

However, each provides a different perspective, depending on which art form is under discussion and the location of the speaker in relation to the subject. While 'Nightingale' is self-centred, spoken by a first-person consciousness as a present, emotional reality and addressed 'to' its subject, 'Grecian Urn' is other-centred and self-effacing, its narrator a quizzical and meditative observer and not, as in 'Nightingale' a suffering subject (an identifiable 'I') participating and implicated in the action. The drama is enacted in the representations of characters on the urn's frieze. Titled 'On', it describes the art object, and its final lines could be interpreted as inscribed upon the urn, like a motto, epigram or message. What is being meditated upon is a static artefact combining properties of narrative painting and sculpture. Ian Jack considered it unlikely that Keats consistently had a particular urn in mind, especially since the poem alludes to details from the Elgin marbles, a painting by Titian, and Claude's *Enchanted Castle*. In other words, its primary subject is the nature of pictorial art in general.[77] Moreover, in 'Grecian Urn' Keats is contributing to a debate stemming from G. S. Lessing's *Laocoon* (1766) which, in the words of a recent scholar of intermediality (dealing with relationships between different media, as intertextuality deals with rela-tionships between texts), took as its 'major idea' that 'works of visual art depict the static realm of the spatial area, whereas works of verbal art depict the linear and temporal developments', as can be said also of music.[78] This distinction derived from the age-old, more specific subject of *ekphrasis* based on Horace's '*ut pictura poesis*' and linking poetry to visual art.[79] Keats's exercise is more light-handed and 'conceited' in the Elizabethan sense than the portentous terms from this critical lexicon suggest. Once again in his sights is a different perspective on melancholy, this time as an affliction especially suffered by the historian seeking to recover the past through an ancient art object.

The term 'narrator' is subtly inappropriate to describe the primary speaker (for want of a better word) in 'Grecian Urn', since there is no 'narrative' brought to completion through time, though the fact that there is not becomes a definition of the uniqueness of the art form. No matter how much the speaker desires a sequence with a beginning and end, bookending the 'middle' of a story represented on the frieze, he is frustrated. Given the literal circularity of the sculptured urn and its unchanging state, there is no beginning or end, just a paradoxical state of immobilised motion, implying but not enacting a past and a future, never changing yet ever repeating. As with a piece of sculpture, we can walk around the urn yet never reach its 'end' as we so decisively do in music. This is the central, ekphrastic difference between the two arts, poetry and visual art. The speaker straddles the two realms, by both speaking *about* the urn in poetry from an external point of view, and also speaking *for* the urn, imputing to it something like an internal consciousness. His mode of address is *to* the urn and figures inscribed on it, as though they can hear and reply to his insistent questions, though they never can. Among these addresses to the depictions is an injunction not to grieve – 'Bold lover, never, never canst thou kiss, | Though winning near the goal – yet do not grieve ...' – acknowledging that arrested figures in the realm of art are immune to the condition which they represent, a frustration prevailing in the world of passing time in which desire is all too often thwarted, leaving 'a heart high-sorrowful and cloy'd | A burning forehead, and a parching tongue'. The injunction is wasted on these figures taken out of time, since they can 'feel' nothing. In a similar way, the urn itself seems solidly material, yet it is hollow and has no interior except empty space.

The word 'still' in the opening line, 'Thou still unravish'd bride of quietness' is pivotal but also ambiguous. In the *Annals* version it is followed by a comma indicating that it refers to the urn's immobility (still *and* unravish'd), whereas in *1820* the lack of punctuation indicates the meaning 'not yet ravished' (still unbroken, or impenetrable). By eliminating the comma in *1820*, Keats enhances the possibility of holding both versions in mind at the same time. We find a similar ambiguity of 'stillness' in Shakespeare's passage in *The Winter's Tale*, a work which culminates in a work of art literally coming to life:

> when you do dance, I wish you
> A wave o' the sea, that you might ever do
> Nothing but that; move still, still so,
> And own no other function ...

(4.4.135-8)

The punctuation in the ode also makes a difference in glossing the intriguing word with its latent violence, 'unravish'd' (which genders the urn female), since 'still, unravish'd' would suggest the urn's secret will *never* be penetrated, while 'still unravish'd' can imply that it is *yet to be* violated in the future. This sets up the logic behind the poem, positing differentiated realms of art and life. In the world of art the urn will (barring future breakage) exist forever in its current state, while in the world of 'life' and temporality, the writer and reader will continue to attempt to penetrate its secret by hypothesising a reconstructed series of events represented in the images, an endeavour which James Heffernan suggests is 'an almost violent urge to *make* it speak'.[80] Here we have one aspect of the historian's professional dilemma, seeking to discover within, or impose upon fragments from the past, a sequential narrative linked by causation.

The next line, 'Thou foster-child of silence and slow time', establishes not only the urn's antiquity (a surviving product of arrested time, and an object which potentially will last forever) but also its absence of sound. 'Silence and slow time' are the essential conditions of the past, of history. However, even 'silent' and without a voice, it can, the poet observes, 'express | A flowery tale more sweetly than our rhyme'. But the paradoxical nature and power of art return with,

> therefore, ye soft pipes, play on;
> Not to the sensual ear, but, more endear'd,
> Pipe to the spirit ditties of no tone.

If one sense exclusively operates to the deprivation of others (sight or sound), the 'deceiving elf' of fancy can create the rest in the perceiver's willed act of imagination. The passage also alerts us to the grammatical equivalent of paradox in a set of oxymorons which Wasserman in particular considers central to the ode: unheard melodies, sensual spirit, 'ditties of no tone', movement and non-movement, time and infinity, change and changelessness, mutability and permanence, past and present.[81] The 'flowery tale' which the urn 'express[es]' places it as a 'sylvan historian', preserving, recording and making present the past, through the images pictured on its surface, frozen in living moments. However, as the poem evolves it is the observing speaker who is established as the more relevant 'historian' in seeking to interpret the work, challenged but thwarted in his attempt to bring it back to life.

Michael Ann Holly in *The Melancholy Art* argues that it is the lot of historians, particularly art historians, to be driven by a desire to retrieve that which has been lost in time past:

> We preserve, study, exhibit, and write about the representational past because we cannot let it go. In other words, we suffer from a case of disciplinary melancholy. The objects from the past stand before us, but the worlds from which they came are long gone. What shall we do with these visual orphans? Research is that defense mechanism erected against the recognition that there is very little about them that we can in the end recover other than the immediacy of their being in the present . . . It may be supercilious to suggest that research in art history is in pursuit of something it can never catch, but surely that unknowability is part of its charm.[82]

Holly quotes the French historian Georges Didi-Huberman: 'The grandeur and misery of the historian is that his desire will always be suspended between the tenacious melancholy of the past *as an object of loss* and the fragile victory of the past as an *object of recovery*.[83] Much that Holly says has explanatory resonance when reading 'Ode on a Grecian Urn'. She speaks of art as comprising 'objects whose world is lost but continuously refound in new contexts' (p. xx). 'All historians of visual art confront countless remnants of the past, fragments of time' (p. xx), and in practising 'the elegiac nature of our disciplinary transactions with the past' (p. 6) the aim is 'translating the visual into the verbal' (p. 5); 'It is an activity that promises warm solace but delivers cool distance' (p. 5). This seems almost exactly the terrain of 'Ode on a Grecian Urn', although the poem itself finds space only in a footnote. All the time, the historian is aware that the past, even when witnessed in the immediacy and concreteness of a work of art, is ultimately irrecoverable. This, Holly writes, 'is the distinctive dilemma of the history of art from which we cannot escape, and melancholy is the key that locks us in' (p. 20). She even plays on Keats's verbal ambiguity: '*Still* art *still* matters, and works of art, in their hushed material presence, insistently press us not to let time swallow them up again' (p. 21). In a 'Response' to Holly's book, the historian Hayden White locates this debate over art mainly in the high Renaissance, the time of Burton and of classical recovery or 're-birth', the literary period dearest to Keats's heart:

> ... in the period of classical art, from the Renaissance to modernism, the artwork is conceived (in Hegelian fashion) to be a thing ... that exists nowhere in history or even within time and space. Which means that the artwork cannot be 'at home' anywhere, but is essentially 'cast out,' banished from human concourse, in a word, abjected. On such a view, the 'history' of art or, at least, the history of the art of the classic type, would have to be imagined as a story of successive failures of ideal actualization. A melancholy story indeed and properly cast in the tones, tinctures, and modalities of a triumph of darkness over light, of power over beauty, and, at the end (of this kind of art), of death over life.[84]

The literary historian's version of melancholy is captured in the memorable opening sentence of Stephen Greenblatt's *Shakespearean Negotiations*: 'I began with the desire to speak with the dead', though his doleful coda is that all he could hear was his own voice.[85] Burton does not reserve a special category for the 'melancholy art' of the historian, but he himself demonstrates it, seeking futilely to make the dead live again. In a sense *The Anatomy of Melancholy* is a prime example of such a resurrection, with its copious 'scholarly' references in documenting the ancient body of learning, and in Burton's obsessive revisions to the work, pursuing a completeness which can never be realised. Burton himself, it seems, suffers from the historian's melancholy alongside other variations.

Keats had already anticipated this melancholic effort to retrieve the past in 'Isabella', a work which elegiacally accentuates the loss of a 'pale vision' of the historical past in which Boccaccio had written his 'old tale'. Boccaccio himself had built into his tale an awareness that the events occurred long ago, were preserved in a ballad, and then recuperated for his own present. It is a subtle reminder of art as the result of some distant, semi-forgotten loss which cannot be fully retrieved, a palimpsest. In 'Ode on a Grecian Urn' the poet approaches this subject in a more contemplative and philosophical, but nonetheless elegiac spirit. The Grecian urn as 'sylvan historian' is seen to depict 'leaf-fringed legend' in scenes of human interchange from the past which will now never change, of figures who cannot be stirred into new life, but it is the poet-speaker who is a secondary historian, puzzling over what 'story' is being told. Whimsically, he asks unanswerable questions about the figures shown in relief around the urn, and they are exactly the kind of questions an historian asks of his or her subject of inquiry:

> What men or gods are these? What maidens loth?
> What mad pursuit? What struggle to escape?
> What pipes and timbrels? What wild ecstasy?

'Struggle to escape' is the first hint that the timeless image may record not only a happy moment, had it existed in time, but also a maddening bafflement since it does not. The fate of the lovers immobilised at their instant of happiness is that they can never consummate their love nor even kiss, no matter how close their lips are, 'Though winning near the goal'. Consolation for the melancholy implication is openly admitted by the whimsical thought,

> yet, do not grieve;
> She cannot fade, though thou hast not thy bliss,
> For ever wilt thou love, and she be fair!

Happiness 'for ever', perhaps, but not happiness here and now which, if replicated in living time by animated lovers, would if nothing else be insatiably exhausting:

> For ever warm and still to be enjoy'd,
> For ever panting, and for ever young;
> All breathing human passion far above,
> That leaves a heart high-sorrowful and cloy'd,
> A burning forehead, and a parching tongue.

De Almeida describes 'For ever panting' as indicating a quasi-medical condition, 'self consumptive love', the torment of 'relentless unconsummation' which romantic medical thinkers 'recognized as the particular terminal symptom of the exhausted but unnaturally excited consumptive patient'.[86] However, as with much of the ode, an ambiguity hangs over whether the condition applies to the images or to our imposed world of 'breathing human passion' which the gods and mortals are 'far above'. The emotional discrepancy between figures captured in a moment of time but existing out of time, is a facet of the historian's melancholy, an inability to discover a definite before-and-after train of causation which could answer the poet's interrogations. Pictorialised, the scene from the past is ever-present, yet because the past is past, it can never reveal the very secrets which the historian wishes to know. A 'mysterious priest' is leading a heifer to sacrifice at an altar, but who are the figures and what is the reason for the sacrificial ceremony they are about to enact? Where do they come from, 'What little town'? Is it 'by river or sea shore', or is it 'Mountain-built'? And with the unsatisfied curiosity driving the historical interrogation and imagination further, comes a projected sympathy even for the invisible, neglected setting, a form of melancholy insight in itself, for the village is left lonely now, 'emptied of this folk' which will never return to their homes:

> And, little town, thy streets for evermore
> > Will silent be; and not a soul to tell
> > > Why thou art desolate, can e'er return.

The word 'desolate' is as strong as 'forlorn' in 'Nightingale', matching the emotional tone of the heifer 'lowing at the skies', which seems to know it is about to die, but never will.

From viewing the 'brede | Of marble men and maidens overwrought | With forest branches and the trodden weed' as part of an unexplained narrative with an imputed time scheme, the poem ends by withdrawing, and instead seeing the Greek vase from the outside, now addressing it in terms of its status as an historical work of art – 'O Attic shape! Fair attitude' – returning to its stillness and antiquity as characteristic of an unchanging object which will last into 'eternity': 'Thou, silent form, doth tease us out of thought | As doth eternity: Cold Pastoral!'. 'Cold' also adds a range of tones, not only physically in temperature but emotionally ungiving in refusing to answer our questions. The time scheme now is the poet's, speaking for all observers in the future, who themselves will pass away:

> When old age shall this generation waste,
> Thou shalt remain, in midst of other woe
> Than ours, a friend to man, to whom thou say'st,

"Beauty is truth, truth beauty,– that is all
Ye know on earth, and all ye need to know."

Punctuation again creates a famous textual *crux*,[87] since in *1820* the quotation marks allow us to hear the whole two lines as 'spoken' by the urn itself, while in the *Annals* version they encircle only the phrase 'Beauty is truth, truth beauty', as though it is a motto emblazoned on the urn. In isolation, this phrase is a rewording of the Neoplatonic adage, 'It is through beauty that we know truth (or virtue)', though adding a corollary to form a kind of *chiasmus*: 'through truth we know beauty'. If the following phrases are also attributed to the urn, then they act as a kind of reproof to historians ('all *ye*', not 'all *we*') who search for more than the record can supply, but if they are the words of the poet then they are more like a resigned admission that the work of art can never supply answers to our questions. As Wasserman puts it, for all the 'apparently clear abstractions' of the urn's motto, they are an '*ignis fatuus*', 'unable to make it give up a meaning that the total poem justifies'.[88] In both cases, a sharp division is created between the temporal world in which the historian lives and operates, and a higher order world of the objects of study, 'all breathing human passion far above', impervious to the operation of time and thus eternal. It is the difference between reality and representation wittily exemplified in Magritte's famous painting with its own equivalent of a 'speaking' work of art, 'Ceci n'est pas une pipe'. The 'need' to know is equally teasing, since it can mean either that we must simply be content with, at best, half-knowledge of the world represented in art, or it can suggest that we can know the important visible component, beauty, as the ultimate 'truth' to be gleaned from an aesthetic object, making the rest unimportant. Does the ode express dismay at what is lost and can never be retrieved, or consolation that at least the most significant 'truth' of beauty will never be lost? Both ways of reading (and many more) return us to Holly's description of the 'melancholy' task of the art historian who, although forced to accept that 'the past is irrecoverable', yet believes that the object of scrutiny is 'so vivid, so tantalizingly concrete' that we are constantly driven to 'repair the damage by ascribing new meanings in the present'. It is equally the self-defeating, melancholy fate of the literary historian, striving to supply meanings and repair *lacunae* in 'Ode on a Grecian Urn' itself. However much a 'friend to man', the object of scrutiny remains unwilling to yield up all its own tantalising secrets, and instead 'dost tease us out of thought | As doth eternity'. All we can do in response is remain 'capable of being in uncertainties, Mysteries, doubts, without any irritable reaching after fact & reason . . .'.

'Ode to Psyche'

It seems a difficult task to extract melancholy from the sustained celebratory tone of 'Ode to Psyche', and at first sight we might assume that Keats included the poem for what he saw as its satisfying poetic quality:

> The following Poem – the last I have written is the first and only one with which I have taken even moderate pains – I have for the most part, dashed of[f] my lines in a hurry – This I have done leisurely – I think it reads the more richly for it and will I hope encourage me to write other thing[s] in even a more peaceable and healthy spirit.[89]

'A more peaceable and healthy spirit' might be contrasted with the poems dealing overtly with illnesses related to melancholy, like 'Lamia', 'Isabella', 'La Belle Dame', and those indirectly related such as 'Ode to a Nightingale' and 'Ode on Melancholy'. We might also conclude that his purpose was based on a kind of intellectual joke, noting that the story's main source, Apuleius' *The Golden Ass*, came too late in classical history to be canonised:

> You must recollect that Psyche was not embodied as a goddess before the time of Apuleius the Platonist who lived after the A[u]gustan Age, and consequently the Goddess was never worshipped or sacrificed to with any of the ancient fervour – and perhaps never thought of in the old religion – I am more orthodox tha[n] to let a hethen Goddess be so neglected –

Not only was Psyche unhailed 'with any of the ancient fervour' because she came so late in classical times – 'O latest born and loveliest vision far | Of all Olympus' faded hierarchy' – but also because Mary Tighe's neo-Spenserian narrative retelling of the whole story, *Psyche; or, the Legend of Love*, which Keats initially admired, had come recently ('lately') in his own lifetime (1809). In the ordering in *1820* there is a further playful touch, obliquely alluding to Shakespeare's King Lear addressing his youngest daughter, Cordelia: 'But now our joy, | Although our last and least, ... what can you say to draw | A third more opulent than your sisters? Speak',[90] suggesting a Keatsian competition between 'Nightingale', 'Grecian Urn' and 'Psyche' as the third in line. It can be seen as offering a resolution to the paradoxes in the first two, showing poetry to be a medium for overcoming the melancholy of the goddess's obscurity.

The wide popularity of Tighe's poem at the time allowed Keats to take for granted that readers would know Psyche's distressing backstory, allowing him, in William A. Ulmer's words, to present the ode as showing 'the mind's capacity to triumph over suffering'.[91] Tighe's dominant tone is undoubtedly melancholic. Her version foregrounds the unremitting misery of Psyche as she is envied, persecuted and humiliated by Venus, until finally pitied and immortalised by Jupiter. On almost every page of her long poem, Tighe draws attention to the 'tender suffering soul' (p. 180) of the heroine, with lines like 'vexed by cares and harassed by distress' (p. 180), and 'Her fate forlorn in silent anguish mourned' (p. 196). By contrast, Keats's snapshot of a rare moment of tranquilly fulfilled love realised in the amatory union of Psyche and Cupid, the soul and *eros*, seems to divert attention from Psyche's misfortunes, and picks up Tighe's challenge in her last stanza of the poem:

> Dreams of Delight farewel! Your charms no more
> Shall gild the hours of solitary gloom!
> The page remains–but can the page restore
> The vanished bowers which Fancy taught to bloom?
>
> (p. 209)

Whereas Tighe leaves her poem and heroine 'Consigned to dark oblivion's tomb', Keats seems intent on answering in the affirmative her rhetorical question, 'can the page restore | The vanished bowers which Fancy taught to bloom?'. He is saying, 'Yes, I will be thy priest . . .', by calling upon Fancy and imagination to bring flowers to fruition.

Whether or not Keats consciously thought about it at the time of composition, 'Psyche' can be said to follow logically on 'Grecian Urn' since it explores another angle of the historian's task in attempting to retrieve and revive the past. Moreover, if we read with the ordering of the 1820 volume in mind, we can find in 'Ode to Psyche' further reflections on melancholy and affinities with its neighbouring poems. Various suggestions along these lines have been offered. Helen Vendler, for example, interprets the poem as concerned with 'healing' the past, in terms of its recuperation of a Psyche lost from history, as Keats seeks to rescue and retrieve the goddess from both neglect and banishment. She affirms it as a poem intended to 'heal its wounds of loss'.[92] The loss is all the more poignant because Keats picks up the story at a point before Psyche has had immortality conferred:

> Fairer than these, though temple has thou none,
>   Nor altar heaped with flowers,
> Nor virgin-choir to make delicious moan
>   Upon the midnight hours;
> No voice, no lute, no pipe, no incense sweet
>   From chain-swung censer teeming;
> No shrine, no grove, no oracle, no heat
>   Of pale-mouthed prophet dreaming.

The intensifying rhetoric of 'none . . . nor . . . no . . .' to be repeated later draws attention to Psyche's uncelebrated, neglected and obscure existence, even in a moment of apparently post-coital fulfilment.

Taking another tack, H. W. Garrod identifies the figure of Psyche as symbolic: 'The open window and the lighted torch – they are to admit and attract the timorous *moth-goddess*, who symbolizes melancholic love'.[93] Garrod's view was doubted by some at the time and it does seem more likely that the 'timorous' woman is confined and destined to wait for Cupid to enter,[94] yet a later critic, John Jones, found Garrod's main point true enough to the poem's spirit. He notes that 'The Greek word Psyche means both "soul" and "moth" or "butterfly"', and points out that in the poem both Cupid and Psyche have 'pinions' or wings. (It is more likely that the reference to her as 'dove' is intended as an endearment rather than a description, though Jones does not address this point.) There is also a significant anticipation of 'Ode on Melancholy' which links the 'death-moth' with 'Your mournful Psyche', the latter serving to emphasise Tighe's more conventional association of Psyche with melancholy.[95] However, positive as the tone is, the poem is not quite devoid of emotional ambiguity, since the poet resolves to 'build a fane | In some untrodden region of my mind, | Where branched thoughts, *new grown with pleasant pain* | Instead of pines shall murmur in the wind' (my italics). Burton, writing of melancholy in general, cites many examples of oxymoronic 'pleasant pain', for example, 'Even in the midst of laughing there is sorrow', 'even in the midst of all our feasting and jollity . . . there is grief and discontent . . . and with a reciprocalty [sic], pleasure and pain are still united, and succeed one another in a ring' (Book I, Sect. I, Memb. I, Subsect. V). Again, though little more than a hint in 'Psyche', the theme of such mixed melancholy will not only return later in 'Ode on Melancholy', but more immediately it is informed by the experiential prevarications in the two previous odes in which pleasure is explicitly mixed with pain. In turn 'Psyche' also introduces the next few poems which directly contemplate conjunctions of pleasure and pain. A very simple transition which we shall look at below is that the final verse leads straight on to the next poem, 'Fancy' presented as a liberated and liberating spirit, as well as picking up the thought in 'Nightingale': 'Adieu! The fancy cannot cheat so well | As she is fam'd to do, deceiving elf'. The emotional staging of the static scene in 'Psyche' is integrated with the poems before and after, as though the ode's placement here in the collection augments the sense that it 'reads the more richly' not only alone but in this new context, illuminated by its neighbouring poems.

Apparently disagreeing with this judgment, Jack Stillinger offers the opinion that 'Psyche' is 'the least easy [ode] to integrate with the others in any unified view'. But in saying so, he apparently inadvertently reveals another similitude evident in the collection as a whole. 'It is', he says, 'more than anything else, a poem about mental life in the modern world … it is up to the poet himself to compensate for the cruel banishment of fairies, gods, myth, and religion by Lockean and Newtonian "cold philosophy"'.[96] Does this not turn the ode into an answer to the apparently intractable problem addressed in 'Lamia'? 'Ode to Psyche' suggests a counterweight to the brutally demystifying rationality of the philosopher Apollonius, who destroys beauty by seeing it merely as a trick or illusion concealing inner ugliness. In 'Psyche' we are offered a different model of the mind (reason, brain, nonmaterial soul, and imagination),[97] as creative and sustaining – 'Beauty is truth' in this case – not the deadening hand of scientific analysis and 'consequitive reasoning'. In 'Psyche', the mind ('psyche' as mental state), beautiful in its own right, 'putting aside numerous objections' from reality, is transformed into a substantial and complete 'soul' when conjoined and complemented with the corporeal 'Sensations' offered by Cupid – the mind which will 'let the warm love in' – driven not by a search for coldly objective truth but animated by feelings. Vendler, anticipating Stillinger's phrase, 'mental life in the modern world', puts this another way, suggesting that the poet is 'purifying himself of sceptical modernity (the dull brain that perplexes and retards) …'.[98] The main part of the poem dwells not so much on the scene with its figures, but more with the willed triumphalism and self-assertion of the poet who is able to defy 'the dull brain'. It provides an antidote to some of the melancholy dilemmas of temporal existence raised in the earlier poems.

'Ode to Psyche' also draws on the invigorating kind of creative melancholy governed by Saturn, analysed by Klibansky, Panofsky and Saxl as 'divine frenzy' and 'the purest and highest power of thought', combining functions of both intellect and soul.[99] This is announced in the anthem-like confidence of the poet speaking as bard, performing the act of immortalising the figure newly initiated into the status of a goddess, by inserting his role into the near-repetition catalogue of deficiencies which are now fulfilled by the poet:

> I see, and sing, by my own eyes inspir'd.
> So let me be thy choir, and make a moan
> Upon the midnight hours;
> Thy voice, thy lute, thy pipe, thy incense sweet
> From swinged censer teeming;
> Thy shrine, thy grove, thy oracle, thy heat
> Of pale-mouth'd prophet dreaming.

With its religious imagery, the ode enacts and celebrates the healing and recuperative power of poetry over melancholy, underpinning a refrain which will, from here on, run through the rest of the poems in the volume, the suggestion that cure of melancholy can be effected by the creative force of poetry. The work of the poet is to construct an alternative reality in the world of self-consistent, ever-fertile plenitude available to his own mind through the imagination:

> And in the midst of this wide quietness
> A rosy sanctuary will I dress
> With the wreath'd trellis of a working brain,
> With buds, and bells, and stars without a name,
> With all the gardener Fancy e'er could feign,
> Who breeding flowers, will never breed the same.

Obliquely, Keats is here echoing the idea behind Shakespeare's Chorus in *Henry V* speaking of the creative imagination as 'the quick forge and working-house of thought' (5.1.Chorus.23), though changing the metaphorical poet from hammering blacksmith to nurturing gardener. It is here that Keats expands the notion of the soul to include other mental faculties such as the 'brain' (reason or thinking process), and 'fancy' (imagination), locating these in the poet-figure who is 'creating' Psyche as a goddess to be worshipped. And 'However, it may be, O for a Life of Sensations rather than of Thoughts!', since 'Psyche' is linked with the preceding odes through conscious reference to the senses. If 'Nightingale' explores the paradoxes of the sense of sound and 'Grecian Urn' of sight, then 'Psyche' incorporates references to all the senses as if in summary inclusiveness, adding touch ('Their lips touched not but had not bade adieu'), and smell ('incense sweet | From chain-swung censer teeming'). For gustatory delights we need to return to Porphyro's exotically delicious feast in 'St Agnes', and forward to 'Ode on Melancholy' where the poet can 'burst joy's grape against his palate fine' and 'taste the sadness' of melancholy's might. At many levels, 'Ode to Psyche', placed centrally and transitionally in the collection, points backwards and forwards to other poems, as though explaining the creative process that has brought them all into being.

'Fancy'; 'Ode' ['Bards of passion and of mirth']; 'Lines on the Mermaid Tavern'; 'Robin Hood'

Although it is hazardous to describe any poems in such a rich and concentrated volume as 'minor', yet these four can be considered as a group, since they are lighter in tone than the others, *jeux d'esprits* consolidating in more lighthearted vein the intellectual playfulness of the previous three odes, and buffering the two more 'serious' odes to follow. They also all deal with different aspects of the kinds of cultural loss and recovery raised in 'Psyche'. They were written in 1818, before the more ambitious 1819 poems in this volume, thereby recapturing a part of Keats's own history, just as they thematically recuperate earlier, Elizabethan literary times, and as 'Isabella' recreates medieval Boccaccio and 'Grecian Urn' and 'Psyche' retrieve ancient mythology. They share common themes that include mixed emotions of melancholy and joy, nostalgia, and satisfaction in bringing back into existence 'lost' dead poets and the ethos of Robin Hood legends. These poems are 'speaking to the dead' by asserting still-living qualities of poets of old. When seen as part of the evolving sequence in the 1820 volume, despite their cheerful tone they take on new significance as more pessimistic meditations on literary fame and its proximity to worldly poverty. Keats had become emotionally burdened and acutely depressed by this perception of the past when he visited Burns' cottage and tomb: 'All is cold Beauty; pain is never done'.[100] Taken together, the poems have strong associations with Milton's 'L'Allegro' and 'Il Penseroso', which had been in Keats's mind when he first composed the poems, since he mentions the phrase 'the Cherub Contemplation' from 'Il Penseroso' in the earlier letter to Reynolds in which he had transcribed the third and fourth poems.[101] In the next sentence of his letter, he mentions Shakespeare's picture of the 'melancholy' Jaques '"under an oak &c"' from *As You Like It*, in which the forest of Arden evokes the world of Robin Hood:

> They say he is already in the Forest of Arden, and a many merry men with him; and there they live like the old Robin Hood of England. They say many young gentlemen flock to him every day, and fleet the time carelessly as they did in the golden world.
>
> (1.1.111–15)

The four poems hang together as a group, and refer back and forth to others in the volume, presenting similar themes in different keys.

The positioning of these four poems together, *seriatim* in the collection, reveals an internal shift of poetic style and mode. Neil Fraistat suggests that despite their apparent modesty, they are positioned as they are because 'they form a climax, a turning point begun at the "Ode to Psyche"';[102] or even earlier, since 'Fancy', for example, picks up the references to fancy in 'Nightingale' and 'Psyche'. Arguably, in imagery and attitude they also turn in different ways towards 'To Autumn' and 'Ode on Melancholy'.

Although pointing fore and aft, they are also a different kind of poetry from the enveloping odes, replacing the poetics of imagination with a poetry of 'Fancy', in which the unburdened surface is expressed with a skimming 'delight and freedom' in Keats's own phrase.[103] The poems seem to have been written as a series, described by Keats as 'specimens of a sort of rondeau which I think I shall become partial to – because you have one idea amplified with greater ease and more delight and freedom than in the sonnet'.[104] In 'Fancy' the *rondeau* is enacted in a series of 'roundings' that keep circling back to repeated lines such as, 'At a touch sweet Pleasure melteth' and 'Oh, sweet Fancy! Let her loose', and a thematic concentration on oscillations between positive and negative thoughts. It seems to me possible that ringing in Keats's mind, as one source and inspiration, was Shakespeare's 'Song' in *The Merchant of Venice*, with its *rondeau*-like form, rhyming trochaic quadrameters, its stated subject of fancy, and its own oscillations between the heart and head, the cradle and the grave:

Tell me where is Fancy bred,
Or in the heart, or in the head?
How begot, how nourished?
[Reply, reply.]
It is engend'red in the eyes,
With gazing fed, and Fancy dies
In the cradle where it lies:
Let us all ring Fancy's knell,
I'll begin it. Ding, dong, bell.

(3.2.63–72)

'Fancy's knell' is rung in the elegiac thought behind the way the poems eulogise dead poets in mock-elegiac fashion, as though poetry has passed away from the modern world.

'Fancy' builds upon the poetic inspiration of 'Ode to Psyche', freeing the creative imagination to 'roam'. The associations with the preceding poem continue:

Then let winged Fancy wander
Through the thought still spread beyond her:
Open wide the mind's cage-door,
She'll dart forth, and cloudward soar.

The 'winged Fancy' recalls the 'winged Psyche', 'thought' refers back to the 'untrodden region of my mind', while the image 'Open wide the mind's cage-door' is a reminder that the 'casement ope at night' of 'Psyche' can let an occupant out in liberation as well as in: 'O sweet Fancy! Let her loose'. There is an emphasis on the frequent contiguity between pleasure, pain and loss that runs through the whole volume: 'At a touch sweet Pleasure melteth' as 'Summer's joys are spoilt by use'; the enjoyment of spring 'Fades as does its blossoming'; while autumn's 'red-lipp'd fruitage . . . Cloys with tasting'. With Fancy presiding 'with a mind self-overaw'd', winter reveals its own pleasures: 'She will bring, in spite of frost, | Beauties that the earth hath lost'. Repeating several times more the circling progression through summer's flowery fertility to autumn with its 'Distant harvest-carols clear; Rustle of the reaped corn', the emerging theme is the constant cycle of sensory gain and loss represented by the fancy encountering fluctuating and mingled experiences – 'She will mix these pleasures up' – in a pattern where opposites, like day and night, are mutually complementary. This synthesising vision is applied first to the natural world, in language resembling John Clare's vignettes of nature ('Freckled nest-eggs', 'rooks with busy caw, | Foraging for sticks and straw'), then to community ('The ploughboy's heavy shoon', 'Sit thee by the ingle, when | The sere faggot blazes bright'), and to human feelings: 'Where's the cheek that doth not fade. | Too much gaz'd at?' . . . 'Where's the eye, however blue, | Doth not weary?'.

There are subtle changes in modes of address adopted in each poem in the volume, and although Aristotle was probably not in Keats's mind, the changes can be suggestively described in the ancient's terminology. Aristotle in his *Poetics* had proposed three genres or literary forms: epic, lyric, and dramatic. Each is distinguished by a different voice and poetic stance. Epic uses third-person narration as the poet tells a story to the reader, lyric is first-person expression of personal feelings, drama has no single narrator or 'self' but projects into the feelings of several characters who 'speak for themselves'. Whether by conscious design behind his chosen sequence of poems, or instinct, or mere accident, Keats's volume follows a similar progression. 'Lamia', 'Isabella' and 'The Eve of St Agnes' are third-person narrative poems, the Elizabethan form of 'minor epics', as the poet tells his tale and guides the reader's responses. 'Ode to a Nightingale' is unequivocally lyric, where the voice is that of the 'sole self' of the poet. Both 'Ode on a Grecian Urn' and 'Ode to Psyche' are also lyrics but with differences in stance, since in both the speaker is in the position of an interlocutor addressing respectively the urn or Psyche, rather than addressing the reader directly; interrogating (the urn) or celebrating (Psyche). In the next four, short poems with which we are dealing here, the point of view is more indeterminate again, and shading into the dramatic mode. There is no true first-person or lyric 'I' among them, but instead a more generalised, exhorting address, as though we are being guided by a bardic commentator to share the thoughts of others. 'Fancy' marks a transition from 'Psyche', where the poet steadily internalises the creative imagination into 'some untrodden region' of the 'mind', towards a point where the poem speaks for or on behalf of the creative 'fancy' itself. 'Ode' ('Bards of Passion and of Mirth'), 'Lines on the Mermaid Tavern', 'Robin Hood', in keeping with their subject matter of earlier drama, could well have been spoken by characters in a play, or at least by fictional *personae* in dialogue with each other. Further, the poems respond to each other as though in dramatic dialogue, and this may partially explain why 'Song of Four Faeries: Fire, Air, Earth, Water' was originally, if somewhat inexplicably, intended for inclusion in *1820*. It is written as a sustained, dramatic dialogue between the four elemental 'characters' which could have complemented the four poems in this group. The chameleon-like drama of 'To Autumn' is emerging.

'Bards of Passion and of Mirth' and 'Lines on the Mermaid Tavern' were by far the earliest in dates of composition, both about 3 February, 1818 when Keats was writing *Endymion*. This suggests that their inclusion in *1820* was for reasons of relevance to the volume in terms of subject and theme, rather than for quality – indeed, John Barnard says that they are 'markedly inferior to the other poetry in the book'.[105] (This in itself adds to the mystery of why Keats did not include the vastly superior 'La Belle Dame'.) Barnard describes how they were part of an earlier, politically-tinged, epistolary exchange between Keats and Reynolds, addressing each other as 'Coscribbler[s]', who had shared poems on Robin Hood as 'a nostalgic lament for a lost past'.[106] They are pitting the 'simplicity' of Elizabethans as 'old poets' against what they saw as modern, subjectively inclined and self-referential 'egoists', in particular Wordsworth, Byron, and Hunt. But again, if this were the initial context for their existence, what do they provide *1820* which made them fit into the collection compiled almost two years later? The answer seems to be that the collocation sets up a running conversation within the volume, not only between these three poems but with others too. In this reading, the word 'No!' which begins 'Robin Hood' functions no longer as a disagreement with Reynolds but as a public riposte to the immediately preceding poem, 'Lines on the Mermaid Tavern', which in its turn answers 'Bards of Passion and of Mirth', itself in dialogue with 'Fancy'. In the new context, the poems are in semi-dramatic dialogue with each other.

'Bards of Passion' picks up from 'Fancy' the inclusiveness of poets as recorders of different emotional states, respectively 'Passion' and 'Mirth', analogous to the Miltonic contrast between 'Il Penseroso' and 'L'Allegro'. The conceit this time is that bards exist in two realms simultaneously. 'Double-lived', their bodies are buried on earth, but their souls are immortalised and able to be read in later times through the works they have written. The distinction reminds us of the nightingale, as the bird passes away but the song continues, and sure enough the image appears on cue, as the bards have similarly 'Double-lives in regions new' in their own heaven,

> Where the nightingale doth sing
> Not a senseless, tranced thing
> But divine, melodious truth;
> Philosophic numbers smooth;
> Tales and golden histories
> Of heaven and its mysteries.

In terms of the collection this reflects back on 'Nightingale' as a poem not about a specific bird but on the nature of music and poetry in general. The existence of older bards may be 'on high' but the works they leave are available for others to use: 'On the earth [they] live again' and 'Here, your earth-born souls still speak | To mortals of their little week'. The lesson is the same as the one taught in different ways in the poems in Keats's volume, from 'Lamia' to 'Ode on a Grecian Urn', that the 'earth-born' life is made up of light and dark, of joy and melancholy intertwined, as the 'little week' of mortals is made up of similar contrasts,

> Of their sorrows and delights;
> Of their passions and their spites;
> Of their glory and their shame;
> What doth strengthen and what maim.
> Thus ye teach us, every day,
> Wisdom, though fled far away.

The voice is different but the song remains the same in all the poems in *1820*. In the case of Keats himself, who endured 'the vale of Soul-making', and in light of the future afterlife of his 1820 volume, the 'double-lived' hope was to become a self-fulfilling prophecy for one who longed to be 'among the English Poets' after his death.[107]

'Lines on the Mermaid Tavern' develops the preceding concentration on deceased 'bards', and also introduces the next poem by referring to Robin Hood. Although the slightest of the three, it continues artfully the vein of a conversation between poems, this time evincing a spirit of intertextual sociability among poets from different generations. The 'Souls of poets dead and gone' are not in 'heaven' but envisaged as still carousing in the Mermaid Tavern, which was especially associated with the Elizabethan poets. The rhythms seem to become comically tipsy as they quaff Canary wine and eat venison pies. 'Robin Hood', although superficially still joking, closes the four 'bardic' poems in more plaintive and elegiac spirit, as though 'Jesting, deep in forest drear'. In the new context, the opening lines of the first two stanzas dismiss the possibility of resurrecting the old poetry: 'No! those days are gone away' and 'No, the bugle sounds no more'. Despite the jaunty rhythm and emphatic tone, the imagery is decidedly melancholy, with hours and minutes 'old and gray' buried under the 'down-trodden pall | Of the leaves of many years'. Sounds of convivial recreation are replaced by silence. It is futile to search for Robin Hood and his band, for 'you never may behold' them, either in their green world or in the tavern of a 'fair hostess Merriment'. 'Gone' is 'the merry morris din' and the heroes of old brought to life by poets. In their place is a bleak contemporary landscape, where, if Robin and Marian could somehow return, they would find a world irrevocably changed for the worse: 'She would weep, and he would craze'. Among other things, these free-spirited, nature-loving socialists would find, as had Lycius and Lamia, that the modern capitalist world requires cash to pay the rent:

> She would weep that her wild bees
> Sang not to her – strange! that honey
> Can't be got without hard money!

In the original context of the letters exchanged by Keats and Reynolds (explaining why the poem is dedicated to 'A Friend'), this verse was part of their ongoing discussion about poetry, contrasting the 'simplicity' of Elizabethan poetry with the kind of conservative Regency literary politics reflected in Hazlitt's critical and pessimistic view. However, in the new context of *1820* we recall more general reverberations of the dismayed transition in 'Nightingale' as the poet is tolled back to his sole self with the word 'forlorn' (lost), as well as the bleak endings of 'Lamia' and 'Isabella', and the final stanza of 'The Eve of St Agnes'. Even the gentler tone of 'Ode on a Grecian Urn' is recalled, since the poems once again reveal the historian's melancholy on realising the impossibility of fully re-entering or recapturing the past. The urn's spoken valediction chimes with the last stanza of 'Robin Hood' in a spirit of reluctant acceptance of irrecoverable loss – 'So it is' – the only recourse being to 'honour' the world of poetry, stories and old heroes, while allowing it to rest in peace in its other world untainted by the present. The two last lines are also re-contextualised in a curious way since, if we put aside the youthful correspondence between Keats and Reynolds, we find a more immediate and serious interpretation informed by the preceding poems. 'Though their days have hurried by | Let us two a burden try' seems to suggest that in this volume the poet, now in collaboration with his reader ('us two'), will venture just two more attempts to come to terms with the melancholy of loss, a task which has so far proved richly elusive.

'To Autumn'

It is easy to understand why almost every critical account of 'To Autumn' begins by quoting Keats's words to Reynolds on returning from London to Winchester, describing the season: 'Really, without joking, chaste weather – Dian skies – I never lik'd stubble field so much as now – Aye better than the chilly green of the spring . . .'. It is especially significant since he continues, 'this struck me so much on my Sunday's walk that I composed upon it'.[108] The result is the ode, and anthologists and critics are accustomed to ascribe its mood of peace and serenity simply to his appreciation of the sights and sounds on a balmy autumn day. However, as usual in Keats's multilayered mind, his emotional state at the time was not so single-noted. Some have detected a political perspective stirred by having just heard the radical speech in London by Henry 'Orator' Hunt,[109] and by having read a series of articles in *The Examiner* linking autumn and thoughts of social justice in the period leading towards the massacre at Peterloo.[110] Others, such as Helen Vendler and Geoffrey Hartman[111] have read the ode in the light of literary history, or as do Jerome McGann and James Chandler, in relation to social conditions of the time. Richard Marggraf Turley detects in 'To Autumn' the prevailing culture of suspicion and surveillance that marked post-Waterloo politics in England.[112] Few, however, have read the poem in the context of its placement in the 1820 volume, intended as its penultimate work, written at exactly the time Keats was beginning to consider and plan his collection. In a sense, composition and publication coincide here, in a way they do not for any other poem in *1820*. 'To Autumn', read in this context, again traces processes of loss, experiential evanescence, and hints of mortality weighed against cyclical renewal, now in a warm and accepting spirit. It is conspicuously placed apart from the three other odes and linked instead with the putatively closing 'Ode on Melancholy', a poem which also turns on acceptance, and draws into coalescence painful loss and existential joy in a single vision. If these two poems provide a stationing point on the journey through 'the vale of Soul-making', it looks like the 'Hyperion' project reached towards the next related stage, dying into a new life of universal compassion, as the poet's role becomes more comprehensively akin to the physician's healing power.

The evidence of the letters sent during the fortnight offer a range of personal feelings that are far from serene, suggesting instead a turbulent and intensely 'fretful' period for Keats. He wrote to Reynolds, 'I have given up Hyperion' (his second attempt at the project), and although this is not the last we hear of the planned epic, and despite the news being delivered so laconically and in such a neutral tone, yet it must have been a disappointment to Keats. He elaborates on his confused emotional state:

> To night I am all in a mist: I scarcely know what's what – but you knowing my unsteady and vagarish disposition, will guess that all this turmoil will be settled by tomorrow morning. It strikes me to night that I have led a very odd sort of life for the two or three last years – Here & there – no anchor – I am glad of it.[113]

As usual he is careful to reassure his correspondent with the positive 'I am glad of it', but the cheering qualifications do not ring entirely convincingly in the light of the 'turmoil' of his mood and circumstances. The motivation behind his trip to London was to discuss with their guardian his own financial hardship, the news of the failure of George's American investment, and the looming necessity of a Chancery case which threatened to be as protracted as the future, fictional 'Jarndyce v. Jarndyce' in *Bleak House*. For his pains he was modestly successful in gaining a loan, but more painfully he was reprimanded for choosing to be a poet by Abbey, jokingly (in bad taste). Adding insult to injury, Abbey quoted against him some cynical lines about would-be poets written by Byron, Keats's own *bête noir*. Keats writes to both Reynolds and Brown that he has little commercial confidence in his future as a poet and resolves instead to work for money, not in the 'apothecary-profession'[114] (though he sometimes considered being a ship's doctor), but in a 'literary' occupation such as theatrical reviewing for periodicals. His hopes of seeing *Otho the Great* on the London stage were ebbing, especially since the bankable Kean, his favoured leading man, was heading off to America. It must also have been difficult to avoid worrying about his own ill-health, less than a year after the trauma of Tom's death, though he does not burden his correspondents with details. However, it was during this week that he begins seriously talking to Woodhouse about publishing 'Lamia' and 'St Agnes Eve' (but not at this stage 'Isabella'), and irritating Woodhouse by his refusal to revise the more erotic material in 'St Agnes'. And he was reading, or rereading, Burton's *Anatomy* in which he could have come across the line 'Of seasons of the year, the autumn is most melancholy',[115] a sentiment which must have struck a chord, especially since circumstances facing Keats could hardly have been more inauspicious.

But the extra and perhaps most important clue to Keats's general anxiety lies in a letter he had written a week before on 13 September to Fanny Brawne, but had delayed sending, explaining if not apologising for his failure to visit her in Hampstead:

> Am I mad or not? I came by the Friday night-coach – and have not yet been to Hampstead. Upon my soul it is not my fault. I cannot resolve to mix any pleasure with my days . . . If I were to see you to day it would destroy the half comfortable sullenness I enjoy at present into down[-]right perplexities. I love you too much to venture to Hampstead, I feel it is not paying a visit but venturing into a fire . . . Knowing well that my life must be passed in fatigue and trouble, I have been endeavoring to wean myself from you: for to myself alone what can be much of a misery? . . . I am a Coward, I cannot bear the pain of being happy: it is out of the question: I must admit no thought of it.[116]

The phrases 'half comfortable sullenness', 'perplexities', 'venturing into a fire', 'fatigue and trouble', 'misery', 'the pain of being happy', all bear witness to a mind in turmoil. There are more hints in letters before and after these, but enough has emerged to suggest that, far from feeling serenely at peace, Keats was in a fluctuating state of extreme anxiety about the future and near despair about the present. 'To Autumn' came, no doubt, as a relief or at least distraction (one of Burton's most frequent recommendations for alleviating melancholy), but behind and around it lay emotional 'mists' and general distress. In a very real sense, the poem came as his cure, however temporary, for melancholy. It is for him the equivalent of Hamlet's relinquishment of ominous anxiety:

> Not a whit. We defy augury. There is a special providence in the fall of a sparrow. If it be now, 'tis not to come; if it be not to come, it will be now; if it be not now, yet it will come. The readiness is all. Since no man of aught he leaves, knows aught, what is't to leave betimes? Let be.
>
> (5.2.218–23)[117]

'To Autumn' can be seen as Keats's 'let be' and 'readiness is all' poem, in its spirit of fatalistic acceptance in the face of mounting troubles.

Writing the poem seems at least temporarily to have calmed Keats's own nerves, even if the circumambient 'turmoil' lying behind its composition does not force its way into the poem in any explicit way. This may help to explain why many readers have also found 'To Autumn' itself as in some way emotionally therapeutic. This poem and the next, 'Ode on Melancholy', offer two different remedies for the prevailing melancholia and sense of loss symptomised in other poems in the collection. Helen Vendler, after discussing at length the impressive range of literary sources and references lying behind the ode, moves on to generalise about the poem itself, mentioning the overarching context of *1820*: 'Generically, then, the autumn ode belongs with poems which debate the value of melancholy, of suffering, or at least of a harsher change ...' (p. 236), 'the absence at the heart of things brings us again into the shrine of Melancholy in the very temple of Delight' (p. 259). She describes the healing effect as 'reparatory' and 'restorative', words which she finds so apt that she repeats them ten times in just ten pages (pp. 258–68). It would seem that in 'To Autumn', Keats might have achieved the kind of poetry which he had been yearning for since abandoning medicine, expressed earlier in 'Sleep and Poetry' as '[Poesy] should be a friend | To sooth the cares, and lift the thoughts of man', and later by Moneta in the poem which he had been writing more or less at the same time, *The Fall of Hyperion. A Dream*: 'sure a poet is a sage, | A humanist, physician to all men'. Out of pain comes solace in the 'vale of Soul-making'. Or to place it in terms he had mentioned in 1817 to describe his temperament when he can live in the in projected empathy without the burden of past suffering or anxiety for the future: 'nothing startles me beyond the Moment. The setting sun will always set me to rights – or if a Sparrow comes before my Window I take part in its existence and pick about the Gravel'.[118] The poem has the capacity to 'put to rights' (repair, restore, heal) the reader, as effectively as does the 'setting sun' in a moment of empathy with external existence.

The mysterious process of somehow making felt what is left unstated is a function of poetic stance, style, and implied attitude. The 'voice' of 'To Autumn' is not the lyric 'I' of 'Nightingale' and 'Psyche', and nor is it imputed to the subject as in the 'Grecian Urn' ode. Instead, it is composed in what Keats described as his 'dramatic capacity', entering 'fully into the feeling' of the poem, extending the direction of the transitional middle poems away from lyric subjectivity. It is also an enactment of the quality 'which', he says, 'Shakespeare possessed so enormously ... – Negative Capability, that is when man is capable of being in uncertainties, Mysteries, doubts, without any irritable reaching after fact & reason ...'.[119] W. J. Bate pronounced that 'The poet himself is completely; absent there is no "I," no suggestion of the discursive language that we find in the other odes; the poem is entirely concrete ...',[120] and other critics have agreed, using their own chosen terms. Ian Jack comments succinctly, 'This is not a poem about Keats: it is a poem about Autumn'.[121] Stanley Plumly speaks of 'the perfection of Keats's mode of disappearance into the text'.[122] Some speak of 'impersonality', while Eric G. Wilson says, 'no "I" explores his sorrows and joys. The poet stands to the side, and points to the beauty of the season ...' (p. 142). Vendler writes, 'the position of the reader vis-à-vis the poem is a strange one. The poet is so unconscious of his reader that we have only the choice of becoming him in his apostrophe and losing our own identity'. Or to reverse the distinction, the reader become unconscious of the poet's voice altogether, as though the season itself is speaking (p. 246). William A. Ulmer detects also 'the manner in which Keats's phrases appear dramatically envoiced and work to reflexively create a dramatic speaker, the text's contemplative protagonist . . . "To Autumn" confesses its investment in a drama of the mind . . .'.[123] However, I would add the important qualification that it is not quite the same as dramatic voices of Shakespeare in his plays, but in his poems, such as Sonnet 12 whose opening lines Keats admiringly chose to transcribe in a letter,[124] and whose images hover allusively behind the last stanza of his own poem:

> When lofty trees I see barren of leaves,
> Which erst from heat did canopy the herd,
> And Summer's green all girded up in sheaves,
> Borne on the bier with white and bristly beard

Or it is the voice within a more modern poem which ponders the mysterious woman whose song 'becomes' the sea of which she sings, in Wallace Stevens' most Keatsian work, 'The Idea of Order at Key West'.[125]

The sensory impressionism of 'To Autumn' is primarily a feat of style, and I need not rehearse here the many critical explorations and explanations which could fill a volume, a small mountain to which I have already contributed my suggested analysis.[126] Rather than repeat these in summary fashion, it might be illuminating to link the ode with one of its neglected sources, James Thomson's The Seasons (1727), in which Autumn is greeted with the poet's 'Philosophic Melancholy'. Keats had attended Hazlitt's lecture on Thomson in February, 1818, in which Hazlitt praised him as 'the best of our descriptive poets' because he 'describes the vivid impression which the whole makes upon his own imagination; and thus transfers the same unbroken, unimpaired impression to the imagination of his readers . . . In a word he describes not to the eye alone, but to the other senses . . .'.[127] Thomson writes,

> When Autumn scatters his departing gleams,
> Warned of approaching Winter, gathered, play
> The swallow-people; and, tossed wide around,
> O'er the calm sky in convolution swift
> The feathered eddy floats, rejoicing once
> Ere to their wintry slumbers they retire,
> In clusters clung beneath the mouldering bank,
> And where, unpierced by frost, the cavern sweats:
> Or rather, into warmer climes conveyed,

With other kindred birds of season, there
They twitter cheerful, till the vernal months
Invite them welcome back – for thronging, now
Innumerous wings are in commotion all.[128]

So much of this percolates into 'To Autumn', but transmuted into Keats's richly condensed style. Thomson's lengthy description of the 'swallow-people' leaving for winter (which continues later), while sharing the word 'twitter', is all inferred rather than explicated in Keats's brief 'And gathering swallows twitter in the skies'. Thomson spells out the approach of winter as the reason for the birds' flight 'to warmer climes', but Keats leaves this unspoken and implied, in a kind of conscious avoidance in order to defer the future. Similarly, Thomson looks forward to their return when 'the vernal month | Invites them back', while Keats again pushes the future aside in savouring the moment: 'Where are the songs of spring? | Think not of them, thou hast thy music too'. The sound of 'innumerous wings' is transferred from birds to bees in the first stanza and the 'wailful choir' of gnats in the last. Thomson also writes later an extended reference to the robin red-breast which, deprived of food in winter tamely enters human quarters, and likewise Keats's robin sings now not in open fields but domesticated 'from a garden-croft'. Elsewhere, Thomson speaks of 'The breath of orchard big with bending fruit', in which a 'deep-loaded bough' is hung with pears, and 'The vine too here her curling tendrils shoot'. Keats's boughs carry a 'load' of apples and fruit on 'the vines that round the thatch-eves run'.

Meanwhile, many barely perceptible echoes of other writers lead back to poems, from Shakespeare's sonnets and from Wordsworth, while Nicholas Roe detects 'the true idiom of English'[129] in sturdy Anglo-Saxon vocabulary praised by Keats as distinctively Chattertonian: 'I somehow always associate Chatterton with autumn. He is the purest writer in the English Language'.[130] Ian Jack extends the range of inter-medial references to include visual art in the painterly stasis of the second stanza,[131] and Andrea Henderson (without mentioning 'To Autumn') attributes what she calls 'the aesthetics of ephemerality' to contemporary artists, Constable's philosophy of 'catching the moment' and Turner's impressionism:

> The aesthetic of the ephemeral celebrated this new relation to objects, finding a beauty in their fugitive qualities at the same time that it recognized the pathos inherent in their transience . . . it also gave rise to a peculiarly modern form of melancholy, for attaching oneself to ephemeral objects meant lamenting the very transience that made them lovely.[132]

All these and more contribute to the alchemical distillation of 'To Autumn', and the overall impression that the subject is not the poet's voice and feelings as he contemplates autumn, but the voice of autumn itself with its capacious heritage in poetry, metaphorically 'conspiring' (from the Latin for 'breathing') with representations of the season as 'Close-bosom friend of the maturing sun'.

Underpinning and sustaining the aspects of dramatic stance, 'Negative Capability', sense of inwardness with the season, and stylistic condensation, is a sustained attitude of unconditional emotional surrender to the ephemeral world as it is. Gone is the ardent pursuit of young lovers which has led to disappointment and death in 'Lamia' and 'Isabella', or the bracing dangers of an uncertain future in 'The Eve of St Agnes'. Gone also is the inevitable frustration attending a desire to hang onto the ideal in 'Nightingale' or interrogate it in 'Grecian Urn'. Gone also is the burden of loss in 'Robin Hood' and the group of poems lamenting the Elizabethan writers. 'To Autumn' resists the temptation to allow the elegiac tone to dominate, as it so easily could have. In its place we are given vignettes presented as scenes of dramatised externality, neither struggling against nor struggling to transcend melancholy, but sublimating it into a new, more complex and inclusive mood. Melancholy is incorporated in the vision but prevented from overloading it. By this point in the 1820 volume it is an ever-present companion, but one that sharpens the sense of transience and impending loss which is essential to appreciating the special beauty of the passing seasons in the natural world:

> the inhabitants of the world will correspond to itself – Let the fish philosophise the ice away from the Rivers in winter time and they shall be at continual play in the tepid delight of summer.[133]

In the human world melancholy cannot be 'philosophised' away since it is the element that paradoxically finds meaning and perceives beauty, as steps along the path of 'the vale of Soul-making'. Time is as present as it is in the 'Nightingale' and 'Grecian Urn' odes. 'Autumn' has at least two time-schemes, one passing from morning to afternoon to evening, and the other from midsummer growth to harvest to post-harvest late autumn on the verge of winter, but the sting of time's tyranny is removed by the implicit 'philosophising' away, or acceptance of the elements that threaten the enjoyment of the moment even as it passes. Acceptance of the necessity of passing time and the season's organically cyclical tasks neutralises dismaying changes in 'Nightingale' from ecstasy to despondence, and the historian's melancholy in 'Grecian Urn' of being excluded from the art-work's antiquity.

This and the next poem provide some resolution, or at least closure, to the direction of the volume. 'Autumn' accepts the necessity of time passing and of reality as it is, without trying to avoid or evade these, while 'Ode on Melancholy' turns melancholy into a positive, creative state to be embraced and celebrated, even at the cost of self-annihilation. 'Ode on Melancholy' offers a face-on confrontation with the condition as a creative stimulus and an emotionally driving force, as if it has finally been identified, driven into the open, and named. Melancholy *almost* intrudes in the third stanza of 'Ode to Autumn', with its anticipation of impending winter, its vocabulary of muted loss in 'the soft-*dying* day', 'a *wailful* choir', 'the small gnats *mourn*' (my italics), and in the image of the 'gathering swallows' preparing to follow the sun. In this sense there is no return at the end to the idealisation of plenitude which had opened the poem, since as in all the poems in *1820*, something is lost, as Paul H. Fry points out:

> Even if "To Autumn" were about the harvest, it could scarcely be a celebration of plenty. Amid stubble-fields, dried-up cottage gardens, and sounds that are humanly intelligible only insofar as they seem mournful, a requiem for plenitude, the senses complete the eclipse of the season by turning to the high frequencies of an empty sky.[134]

But the effect is far from depressing because of the inevitability of change. Without post-harvest stubble fields there will be no new growth, and without new growth there will be no harvest, so that the end of the ode points back to its beginning to be re-enacted in the next summer.

Arguably 'To Autumn' loses less of its potential meanings than the others in the collection by being anthologised and read in isolation from the rest, yet it does seem to acquire an extra dimension if seen as the penultimate poem in the volume, offering a 'promised end' of consolation to the book of melancholy. This double-status, as stand-alone monad and companion-piece in a collection, might be explained by the fact that in this one case the writing and the publication coincided. The emerging themes of the other poems are coming to the forefront of Keats's discriminating mind, as though now he has become conscious of the journey undertaken in the earlier poems of the collection, and the insistent presence and diversity of melancholy throughout. Since it was composed shortly before he decided to put together his own anthology and may even have galvanised the idea, it is perhaps not surprising that it should reconcile many of the conflicts raised in the earlier poems. There is something of Burton's most recurrent advice for those suffering from a wide array of different versions of melancholy, to exercise patience, acceptance, and endurance (on a page which Keats marked, though not these words in particular):

if it may not be helped, it must be endured . . . time and patience must end it.
> The mind's affections patience will appease,
> It passions kills, and healeth each disease.

(p. 464)

The healing quality of acceptance is also based partly on the reader's extra-textual awareness that it was Keats's last, great completed poem (with the possible exception of the 'Bright Star' sonnet). In this moving sense it has the quality of a 'rest in peace' and 'let be' moment. But it is not quite the final moment of Keats's encounter with melancholia in the volume.

'Ode on Melancholy'

If 'To Autumn' has a self-effacing persona and a preference for 'indolence', the intrusive speaker in 'Ode on Melancholy' adopts a stance of active agency. The very title suggests a direct confrontation with what, I have argued, is a running theme of the volume, melancholy, now presented in a personified form. In its defiantly affirmative acceptance of the state, and immersion in its emotional paradoxes, the poem celebrates the capacity to turn an apparently negative emotion of melancholy into a state of positive creativity and existential joy, recalling the trajectory of 'Fancy'. Hrileena Ghosh has noted that in defiance of our expectation raised by the word, here melancholy '*heightens* perceptions of reality'.[135] The poem emphatically advises against deadening emotional pain with 'dull opiates' and drowning in melancholy – 'No, no, go not to Lethe' – and instead recommends revelling in the state as a way of celebrating the transience which provokes the feeling. Here we have something closer to 'divine frenzy', the poet-healer asserting a form of melancholy which contains its own antidote, just as Burton had dedicated his life to melancholy as a way of overcoming it. To put it a different way, as does Brittany Pladek, this is the poem which consummates a direction of Keats's thinking, when he 'reoriented his aesthetic and ethical perspective to accommodate a poetry tasked with appreciating pain rather than alleviating it'.[136]

Keats may have been remembering one of his own very earliest poems written in 1814, 'Fill for me a brimming bowl', where he begins by wishing to 'drown my soul' with wine to which is added 'some drug, I To banish Woman from my mind' – 'as deep a draught I As e'er from Lethe's waves was quaffed'. This was written after he had seen a mysterious, hauntingly beautiful woman in Vauxhall; if only she had smiled at him, the poet muses, 'I should have felt "the joy of grief"', a phrase from Thomas Campbell's *The Pleasures of Hope* (1799), showing that Keats already had been contemplating the painfully mixed emotion of melancholy. As it is, the woman is lost to him, but 'Even so for ever she shall be | The Halo of my Memory'.

'Ode on Melancholy' belongs with 'Lamia' as the two most Burtonian poems in the volume, in their cultural heritage from the Renaissance. As Klibansky, Panofsky and Saxl argue, it does not build upon Romantic models of melancholy, but instead scorns these 'with an imperious gesture' in favour of the Renaissance:

> Restless and 'wakeful' the poet feeds his melancholy with all his mind and senses, making it embrace all the bright splendor of created things ... It is no coincidence that this new melancholy, which discovers the sanctuary of the Goddess of Melancholy 'in the very temple of Delight' returns once more to the antithetic precision and mythological extravagance of the great Elizabethans.[137]

It marks a return to Spenserian allegory, Milton's 'Il Penseroso', and Burton's all-inclusive, ambivalent state, and a turning-away from the potential self-indulgence and fetish of Romantic melancholy. Despite its brevity, there is a narrative and an argument in 'Ode on Melancholy', carried by the syntactical progression from 'do not . . .', 'instead [do] . . .', 'because . . .', incorporating cryptically Burton's method of categorising symptoms and cures. It has a definite and end-stopped closure defining the direction of the ordered collection, pointing towards the poet's prophecy of a posthumous apotheosis for his works and life as among melancholy's 'cloudy trophies'. If for no other reason, this could aptly draw to a close his collection.

The 'narrative' had begun in a first stanza which Keats deleted:

> Though you should build a bark of dead men's bones,
> And rear a phantom gibbet for a mast,
> Stitch creeds together for a sail, with groans
> To fill it out, blood-stained and aghast;
> Although your rudder be a dragon's tail
> Long sever'd, yet still hard with agony,
> Your cordage large uprootings from the skull
> Of bald Medusa, certes you would fail
> To find the Melancholy – whether she
> Dreameth in any isle of Lethe dull.

Miriam Allott detects Burton's influence: 'The violent imagery suggests a recent reading of Burton's account – to which K's ode is in effect a reply – of the melancholy that leads to suicide in *The Anatomy of Melancholy*'.[138] Burton mentions hanging oneself, jumping from a high building and plunging a dagger into the heart, and he says suicidal feelings can be caused by many feelings such as 'love, grief, anger, madness and shame'. He describes the state in one of his own poems, whose persona is a sufferer from the 'hell ... found in a melancholy man's heart':

O sad and odious name! a name so fell,
Is this of melancholy, brat of hell.
There born in hellish darkness doth it dwell,
The Furies brought it up, Megara's teat,
Alecto gave it bitter milk to eat.
And all conspir'd a bane to mortal men,
To bring this devil out of that black den.
Jupiter's thunderbolt, not storm at sea,
Nor whirlwind doth our hearts so much dismay.
What? am I bit by that fierce Cerberus?
Or stung by serpent so pestiferous?
Or put on shirt that's dipt in Nessus' blood?
My pain's past cure; physic can do no good. (Book I, Sect. IV, Memb. I)

He concludes, 'all other diseases whatsoever, are but flea-bitings to melancholy in extent ... death alone must ease them'. Keats may have Burton's account in mind and he is certainly addressing suicidal thoughts, but in a quite different spirit. His stanza turned out to be a false start to the poem upon which he was launching. Its imagery is too exaggeratedly Gothic in the most literary sense, with its 'bark of dead men's bones', 'phantom gibbet', with a 'dragon's tale | Long severed' for a rudder and its rigging made from 'large uprootings from the skull | Of bald Medusa', and the effect is closer to heightened parody than the despair of Burton's speaker. These are remnants of the more recent but increasingly outmoded eighteenth century manifestations of poetic melancholy satirised by Peacock, and out of place in Keats's conscious return to the Elizabethans throughout the collection. It is not difficult to see why Keats cancelled it since it hits the wrong note and its final lines are metrically awkward. But it does set up the central direction of the poem, a quixotic task 'To find the Melancholy' which lies beyond death, as it 'Dreameth in any isle of Lethe dull' in the underworld, and to confront it. So we are plunged instead into a process of questing and mythologising.

A different kind of false start, this time deliberate and conceptual, opens the poem as it stands. The first stanza rejects the strategy of seeking Lethe through a death-wish for narcotic oblivion which too 'drowsily' causes self-annihilation:

No, no, go not to Lethe, neither twist
Wolf's-bane, tight-rooted, for its poisonous wine;

Nor suffer thy pale forehead to be kiss'd
By nightshade, ruby grape of Proserpine;
Make not your rosary of yew-berries,
Nor let the beetle, nor the death-moth be
Your mournful Psyche, nor the downy owl
A partner in your sorrow's mysteries;
For shade to shade will come too drowsily,
And drown the wakeful anguish of the soul.

Burton, in the same passage quoted above, in distinguishing 'frenzy' from other kinds of melancholy, had sought 'to separate it from such as accidentally come and go again, as by taking henbane, nightshade, wine, &c' (Book 1, First Partition, First Member, Subsection. IV). Keats had first written 'hensbane' but substituted 'Wolf's-bane' (aconite), possibly to inject a Gothic hint of lycanthropia, one of Burton's more extreme categories of melancholy.[139] It was associated with a range of extreme symptoms, including melancholy, terror, mania, and 'gay delirium'.[140] Henbane, despite the innocuous associations of its name, was just as dangerous since it could induce a sleep close to, or even causing death; it may have been the drug given by Shakespeare's Apothecary to Juliet. All parts of the yew tree, which used to be planted in graveyards to keep animals away, are poisonous, including the seeds of the berries. The 'ruby grape of Proserpine', as queen of the underworld, is the true monarch of Lethe, and Evans tentatively identifies it as 'woody nightshade (*Solanum Dulcamara*), or bittersweet', another danger-ously poison flower found on Hampstead Heath, bearing intensely red fruit.[141] The name itself, joining 'bitter' and 'sweet' summarises the kind of melancholy which is the subject of 'Ode on Melancholy' and some of the other poems in the collection. Keats's precision about 'poisonous wine' extracted from deadly plants dates back to his study of medical botany under William Salisbury's supervision, as well as prompts from Burton.[142] The 'death moth' (or hawk moth) was thought to be an omen of death, and so was the clicking sound of the 'deathwatch beetle', to which Keats had already alluded in *Endymion*: '. . . within ye hear | No sound so loud as when on curtain'd bier | The death-watch tick is stifled'. The accompanying partners, 'mournful Psyche' and 'downy owl', indicate nocturnal suffering in slow death, which comes 'too drowsily' to appreciate or savour 'sorrow's mysteries'. In sum, the stanza warns against a passive, submissive wallowing in the kind of suicidal melancholy which will 'Drown the wakeful anguish of the soul' without consciousness of the effect. It marks a withdrawal from the mood of 'To Autumn' and points to something new, and also as Andrea Henderson argues, the speaker of the poem 'distinguishes his from earlier accounts of melancholy by speaking of it not as a disease but as an experience to be sought'.[143]

The second stanza recommends the alternative route, a 'wakeful' encounter with the emotional state, using it as a means of heightening awareness of the beauty of the ever-changing, natural world:

> But when the melancholy fit shall fall
> Sudden from heaven like a weeping cloud,
> That fosters the droop-headed flowers all,
> And hides the green hill in an April shroud;
> Then glut thy sorrow on a morning rose,
> Or on the rainbow of the salt sand-wave,
> Or on the wealth of globed peonies;
> Or if thy mistress some rich anger shows,
> Emprison her soft hand, and let her rave,
> And feed deep, deep upon her peerless eyes.

However, as the first line of the stanza indicates, the condition cannot really be 'sought' but is experienced by chance when 'the melancholy fit shall fall', almost as a miracle. When this happens it must be seized upon and savoured to the full, in a 'gormandizing' spirit, to use the word Shakespeare applied to the 'surfeit-swell'd' Falstaff (2 *Henry IV*, 5.5.53). The first seven lines employ the associative development of logic through imagery that Keats admired in the sonnets of the 'Whim King', Shakespeare.[144] Melancholy falls as a 'fit' over the sufferer like a cloud, and causes tears as if the cloud is 'weeping' rain; rain refreshes the 'droop-headed flowers all' but it also resembles a veil or funeral 'shroud' obscuring the 'green hill'. So, the poem advocates, melancholy, like rain in nature, can be redefined as a creative force causing the morning roses and 'globed peonies' to flower, and it can create the beauty of the rainbow caused by the waves meeting the sand on a beach. Peonies are the only poisons in this benign medicine chest since they are related to wolfsbane, but de Almeida associates them more specifically with 'true melancholy' as a 'prescription or sign of the way to poetic truth', the name Paeon being an epithet for Apollo in his healing capacity.[145] To 'glut thy sorrow' in an act of gorging is also to redefine the negative state as positive, transforming the 'drowsy' to the 'wakeful' and the life-denying to life-enhancing. Similarly, even the 'rich anger' of a mistress can produce beauty in the sparkle it brings to her eyes. Jennifer Radden describes the central paradox at work, as the poem moves towards its resolution:

> Keats's evocation of these dual aspects of melancholy, this stress on the paradox uniting sensual pleasure, energy, and vitality, on the one hand, and

despair, suffering and passivity on the other, elevates his writing on melancholy to a place beside that of Elizabethan authors.[146]

Much critical debate about whether the mistress is a carnal lover, or the figure that Burton often addresses as 'Dame Melancholy' herself, seems at first initially to be resolved as the former. This particular 'she' is mortal, and the corollary paradox applies, that recognition of mortality induces the awareness of beauty in the perceiver: 'She dwells with Beauty – Beauty that must die'. In this case beauty is not the eternal truth of the work of art, but a precarious and fragile moment, its preciousness enhanced by the knowledge that it will not last. Recalling the earlier poem 'Fancy', pleasure equally is a product of its very transience, always on the cusp of saying goodbye or turning to its opposite even at the moment of its intense enjoyment:

> And Joy, whose hand is ever at his lips
> Bidding adieu; and aching Pleasure nigh,
> Turning to poison while the bee-mouth sips.

This leads to the culmination of the poem's narrative logic, its final, paradoxical discovery, that without melancholy we cannot have 'delight': 'Ay, in the very temple of Delight | Veil'd Melancholy has her sovran shrine', a perception which can be glimpsed only by one – pre-eminently the poet – who is prepared to awaken the senses and embrace melancholy as a vital key to pleasure, and joy as paradoxical stimulus to the emotional pain of melancholy: 'Though seen of none save him whose strenuous tongue | Can burst Joy's grape against his palate fine.' Such an acolyte is both an enlightened devotee and a victim, one of melancholy's helpless but willing 'trophies', as poet and poem coalesce: 'His soul shall taste the sadness of her might, | And be among her cloudy trophies hung'. Here Keats joins Burton in the shrine of melancholy, as fellow trophies to its power.

Were it not so modest in form and scope, the buoyant spirit driving 'Ode on Melancholy' might be likened to weightier works that mark the final, creative output of composers such as Beethoven, Schubert and Mahler, in which the elegiac is subsumed within a defiant spirit that accepts suffering and pain as a positive coalescence and purpose of art. It provides an elegant climax to the volume's varying conceptions of melancholy.

'Hyperion. A Fragment' (An Addendum?)

Although I have argued in Chapter 2 that 'Hyperion. A Fragment' was included in the volume against Keats's wishes, and that it may upset the impression of thematic finality to the volume achieved by 'To Autumn' and 'Ode on Melancholy', yet it admittedly continues to manifest and explore different kinds of melancholy. This is not surprising since the subject had been close to the poet's mind throughout 1818 and 1819 when he was writing the other poems. Some links will be briefly sketched here, and also tentatively related to the post-*1820* fragment, *The Fall of Hyperion. A Dream*. The latter is more focused on what seems to be the next stage of Keats's thinking, considering the poet as physician, healing hurt minds, itself a natural development from *1820* and one of Keats's abiding preoccupations.

The version of the proposed epic, begun in the autumn of 1818 and abandoned in April 1819, had been yeasting in Keats's imagination after completing *Endymion*. He envisaged it as a kind of sequel to that poem, describing it to Haydon on 23 January:

> in Endymion I think you may have many bits of the deep and sentimental cast – the nature of *Hyperion* will lead me to treat it in a more naked and Grecian Manner – and the march of passion and endeavor will be undeviating – and one great contrast between them will be – that the Hero of [*Endymion*], – being mortal, is led on, like Buonaparte, by circumstance; whereas the Apollo in Hyperion being a fore-seeing God will shape his actions like one.[147]

The mortal Endymion had been buffeted by 'circumstances' while Apollo is 'fore-seeing' since his future as a victorious god is revealed to him by Mnemosyne. He does not enter until Book III, and before this Keats embarks on the kind of conscious mythologising that he had practised in 'Ode to Psyche', since the defeated Titans under their leader Saturn and saviour Hyperion had also been a trove of ancient myths neglected and overlooked by scholars and poets preferring tales of the usurping Olympians under Apollo.

The fallen Titans are indeed a picture of the most dejected and despondent kind of melancholy, 'effigies of pain', initially presented through the figure of Saturn, 'quiet as a stone'. His stillness and silence in 'the shady sadness of a vale' is emotional as well as physical, and mirrored in the stasis of the scene:

> Upon the sodden ground
> His old right hand lay nerveless, listless, dead,
> Unsceptred; and his realmless eyes were closed.

Saturn is approached by the goddess Thea, Hyperion's wife, who acts as a sympathetic interpreter of his mourning state. She internalises his feelings, and to that extent enacts a poet's function as an emotional respondent:

One hand she press'd upon that aching spot
Where beats the human heart, as if just there,
Though an immortal, she felt cruel pain:
    . . .
"Saturn, sleep on: – O thoughtless, why did I
"Thus violate thy slumberous solitude?
"Why should I ope thy melancholy eyes?
"Saturn, sleep on! While at thy feet I weep."

Her sympathy is ineffective as a rallying cry to action, and she too is rendered impotently tearful: 'And still these two were postured motionless, | Like natural sculpture in cathedral cavern'. Saturn's chief despair, that he has lost his 'strong identity . . . real self', is couched in terms that align him with a melancholy artist-poet who can no longer create '"Beautiful things made new, for the surprise of the sky-children"': '"But cannot I create? | "Cannot I form? Cannot I fashion forth | "Another world, another universe . . .?"'. Thea leads him back, 'rous'd from icy trance' to the equally despondent Titans. Among these, the only god resisting melancholy is the now ascendant Hyperion, who is instead 'full of wrath', stamping his foot and roaring in rage, berating his colleagues as '"effigies of pain!"': '"O spectres busy in a cold, cold gloom! | "O lank-eared Phantoms of black-weeded pools"'. Urged on by his father Coelus, Hyperion resolves to stir Saturn and the Titans, and lead them to a counter-revolution which will prove ultimately doomed.

It steadily becomes clear that the real direction of this version of 'Hyperion' is away from the stasis of melancholy to the dynamism of change conceived as progress, and a steady chorus of voices proclaims the necessity of leaving the past to create the future as a 'law of nature' voiced by Saturn:

"But eagles golden-feather'd, who do tower
"Above us in their beauty, and must reign
"In right thereof; for 'tis the eternal law
"That first in beauty should be first in might:
"Yea, by that law, another race may drive
"Our conquerors to mourn as we do now".

The future victor, predicted by Clymene 'wording timidly among the fierce', will be '"The morning-bright Apollo! Young Apollo"', the son of Jupiter (himself a son of Saturn) who had triumphed over the Titans, thus establishing the rule of the Olympian gods.

In the unfinished Book III we turn decisively away from the doomed Titans ('O leave them, Muse!') to meet the next generation with the emergence of this protagonist. Apollo as 'the golden theme' is introduced with music, strains of 'the Delphic harp' and 'Dorian flute', and he grows up in a burgeoning natural setting. Olive groves, poplars, palms, beech-trees, lilies, hazel thickets, and nightingales mark him as the young poet heading for ascendancy, not through physical prowess but natural gifts of art. His future destiny is recognised by Mnemosyne, whose double function combines memory of the past and knowledge of the future. Apollo confesses to her his own, inexplicable melancholy:

> For me, dark, dark,
> And painful vile oblivion seals my eyes:
> I strive to search wherefore I am so sad,
> Until a melancholy numbs my limbs.

In the Keatsian allegory of a poet's growth, the young Apollo is passing through his own 'vale of Soul-making', learning by taking upon himself the sufferings of others, not knowing exactly why. He asks her the reason for his state, and although she remains mute he can read her face – 'Knowledge enormous makes a God of me' – and he undergoes a violent change, 'Most like the struggle at the gate of death' which allows him to 'Die into life' ready to metamorphose into a god. It is this encounter between Apollo and Mnemosyne, renamed as the priestess Moneta, which is to open Keats's equally unfinished revision, *The Fall of Hyperion. A Dream*, which was planned to instate him as god of poetry, music, medicine, and the sun. But 'Hyperion. A Fragment' leaves him still on this threshold, and the work is abruptly truncated after two and a half Books of a proposed four (judging from the precedent of *Endymion*, which the 'Advertisement' specifies). It is difficult to see exactly how he planned to proceed with the narrative. Logically it would culminate in a confrontation between Hyperion and Apollo, but such a struggle risks being an anticlimax and even incongruous, given the differences between the wrathful, belligerent Hyperion and the more artistic dreamer-poet, Apollo, with the latter needing to emerge victorious. As Sperry asks, 'Would Hyperion have been brought directly into confrontation with Apollo and been forcibly dispossessed? Or would he have recognized the superiority of his adversary and given way without a struggle?'[148] Perhaps the more pacifist fatalism expressed by Oceanus, whose 'voice is not a bellows unto ire', points the way towards a conclusion: '"We fall by course of Nature's law, not force | Of thunder, or of Jove . . . | Receive the truth, and let it be your balm"'. But we will never know the projected ending, even if Keats himself knew. Because of the indeterminacy, I find myself in less than full agreement with Fraistat, who in a footnote suggests that the ending to 'Hyperion. A Fragment' 'is dramatically appropriate to the volume'.[149] Rather, it seems inconclusive.

A related apparent problem is that in essence the 'Fragment' has already effected the result of the power struggle before it has even taken place, since 'Nature's law' that 'first in beauty shall be first in might' has already been demonstrated or at least anticipated in the words of Oceanus:

> "and our fair boughs
> Have bred forth, not pale solitary doves,
> But eagles golden-feather'd, who do tower
> Above us in their beauty, and must reign
> In right thereof; for 'tis the eternal law
> That first in beauty should be first in might:
> Yea, by that law, another race may drive
> Our conquerors to mourn as we do now".

Despite the melancholia depicted in the Titans' condition, the real theme of the poem seems not to be that state, but revolution and necessary political change as the new defeats the old. Ziegenhagen, adds that this is consistent with many other Romantic-era writings,[150] and Kenneth Muir long ago also proposed revolutionary change as the dominant theme of the fragment.[151] The Titans are emotionally pitiful but not admirable in their misery, and sympathies are flowing away from them towards the more optimistically pictured Apollo by the end of the fragment. The narrative does not allow the summating operation of ecstatic paradox of 'Ode on Melancholy' in which joy and sorrow are fused, since in 'Hyperion' the figures representing melancholy must be superseded and left in the past, as required by the fable. It is relevant also, as Bate, Gittings and Sperry all mention, that Keats's composition of 'Hyperion. A Fragment' was proceeding at the time when Tom Keats died on 1 December, 1818, and that after this he confessed, 'it will take some time to get into the vein again'.[152] Understandably, it seems he never did, and one contributory factor could be that in the circumstances the inherent optimism of the poem's direction could not accommodate the agonised and conflicted feelings he was undergoing, simultaneously grieving for his brother and in love with Fanny Brawne after their 'understanding' was reached on Christmas Day, 1818. It was probably the most emotionally turbulent period in his life, and not a time when he could 'strain [his] ne[r]ves at some grand Poem',[153] especially one which, as Stuart Sperry suggests, 'attempted too ambitious an assimilation of conflicting viewpoints and ideas'.[154]

We shall never know exactly the circumstances surrounding Keats's clear reluctance and the publishers' decision to print 'Hyperion. A Fragment'. We know from the 'Advertisement' that the publishers alone accepted responsibility, 'as it was printed at their particular request, and contrary to the wish of the author', strongly confirmed in Keats's annotation written for Burridge Davenport. However, it is improbable that Taylor and Hessey could smuggle it in without at least his knowledge if not agreement. He must at least have known of the proposed inclusion before publication, and may even have proofread it, though there is no direct evidence of this. Albeit reluctantly, he seems to have ended up accepting the decision.

An obvious reason for Keats's objection was that he had discarded this earlier version before he wrote the best of the poems in *1820*, and in this sense he may have regarded it as outdated or surpassed in terms of his own *oeuvre* by the end of 1819. He had also already proceeded with a radical revision of the epic, eventually to be published posthumously in incomplete form as *The Fall of Hyperion. A Dream*, which most scholars deem superior in quality, and this alone would have provided reason enough for his discomfort with publication of the earlier abandoned draft. His efforts at revision had been concentrated and sustained over a significant period from mid-July to 21 September 1819, so the project of finally publishing an epic on the topic was not idly undertaken but part of the author's longer but still current ambitions. He was, it seems, determined eventually to finish the work once he had resolved the internal stylistic and narrative problems. Stating his literary priorities while writing *Endymion* the youthful poet had asked rhetorically, 'Did our great Poets ever write short Pieces?',[155] and in 'To Charles Cowden Clarke' he had remembered the lesson of his tutor that 'epic was of all the king'. The second date, 21 September, was the very day he had apparently started thinking of the 1820 collection, making it equally understandable that he should put his efforts into this more immediately achievable task. Moreover, and equally cogently, publication of the unfinished work would risk rendering superfluous and potentially unpublishable a future, reconstructed version, should it ever be completed, by losing potential readers who may have seen it as duplication. Keats had 'given up' the second, but this does not necessarily mean he had done with it forever, and although ill and exhausted he could be forgiven for at least hoping for enough time and health to publish his second epic in his lifetime, thus maintaining the career pattern of alternating a collection of short poems and an epic.

However, the reasons for Keats's dismay were probably also aesthetic and thematic, if we are to accept that he wished his collection of poems to end with 'To Autumn' and 'Ode on Melancholy', a pair which, I hope to have shown, provide a neat sense of closure to an integrated, poetically conceived 'anatomy of melancholy'. In this sense, 'Hyperion. A Fragment', whatever its quality and however highly it was judged by contemporary admirers, could be seen as distracting from the achieved finality of the shorter poems, and leading in a related but different direction concerning the capacity of poetry to alleviate human suffering with both words and deeds, which was to be the central enquiry of *The Fall of Hyperion. A Dream*. As it stands, the ending of 'Hyperion. A Fragment' makes no attempt to suggest a resolution, ending mid-sentence in what may be a deliberate exaggeration of its incompleteness, giving Keats a kind of pyrrhic, even petulant victory, by visually suggesting that this is no proper way to conclude a compact, aesthetically and thematically unified collection on the nature of melancholy:

> During the pain Mnemosyne upheld
> Her arms as one who prophesied.– At length
> Apollo shriek'd;– and lo! From all his limbs
> Celestial   *   *   *   *   *
> *   *   *   *   *   *   *   *
>   THE END

It was not really where he had intended to finish his volume, but like Hamlet he decided to 'let be'.

She lives in Beauty - Beauty that must die
And Joy whose hand is ever at his lips
Bidding Adieu; and aching Pleasure nigh
Turning to Poison while the Bee-mouth sips
Aye, in the very temple of delight
  Veil'd Melancholy has her sovran shrine
  Though seen of none but him whose memory
Can burst-joys grape against his palate fine
His soul shall taste the anguish of her might
And be among her cloudy trophies hung

6.2 Keats's manuscript 'Holograph Stanza 3, "Ode on Melancholy"', New York Public Libraries Digital Collections, Henry W. and Albert A. Berg Collection of English and American Literature, IMAGE IDpsnypl_berg_1372. In the public domain.

Notes

1. To Reynolds, 11 July 1819, *LJK*, 2, p. 128.
2. Lowes, 'The lovers maladye of hereos'.
3. Chambers, p. 584.
4. Patterson, p. 185 ff.
5. Chambers, p. 385.
6. Summarised by de Almeida, *Romantic Medicine*, p. 188.
7. Sperry, pp. 293, 294.
8. For associations between the snake and healer Aesculapius, see de Almeida, *Romantic Medicine*, p. 186.
9. William Hazlitt, 'On Gusto'.
10. For example, Bate, *John Keats*, p. 544: 'This new use of myth was to be brisk, objective, detached, and to possess at least some elements of the comic'; Dunbar, 'The Significance of the Humor in "Lamia"'.
11. Chambers, p. 589.
12. Dunbar, p. 21.
13. The point is made by Haley, p. 245.
14. Bennett, p. 174.
15. Hazlitt, *The Complete Works*, V, p. 9.
16. Haydon, 2, p. 72.
17. Keats, *The Complete Poems*, ed. John Barnard, Appendix 5, p. 527.
18. Roe, *John Keats*, p. 336.
19. To Bailey, 10 June 1818, *LJK*, 1, p. 292.
20. Burton, *Anatomy of Melancholy*, Book 2, Sect. II, Memb 1.
21. Quoted by Laura E. Campbell, 'Unnecessary Compromise: Publisher Changes to "Ode to Psyche"'.
22. de Almeida, *Romantic Medicine*, p. 212.
23. Miriam Allott suggests that Keats read the fifth edition (1684) of Giovanni Boccaccio, *The Decameron* (London, 1620), originally printed by Isaac Jaggard and possibly translated by John Florio. Keats, *The Complete Poems*, ed. Miriam Allott, p. 326.
24. Turley, *Bright Stars: John Keats, Barry Cornwall, and Romantic Literary Culture*, esp. pp. 45–53.
25. For the reception of Boccaccio in the Romantic age, see Brand, pp. 110–18.
26. See Haworth, 'Keats's Copy of Lamb's *Specimens of English Dramatic Poets*'.
27. Quotations from Freud, xiv (1914–18), p. 246.
28. To Reynolds, 3 May 1818, *LJK*, pp. 276–8.
29. Ward, p. 174; Stillinger, 'Keats and Romance', p. 598.
30. Matthews, p. 157.
31. To Woodhouse, 22 September, 1819, *LJK*, 2, p. 174.
32. McDowell, p. 23.
33. This suggestion is made in the light of Keats's own later self-evaluation of the poem in *LJK*, 2, pp. 174, 183; and Woodhouse's report in 2, pp. 162–3. Although too long to consider here, the quotations repay consideration.
34. Ricks, p. 146.
35. Eliot, 'Hamlet and his Problems'.

36. Hoeveler, 'Decapitating Romance: Class, Fetish, and Ideology in Keats's *Isabella*'.

37. Burton, *Anatomy*, 'Democritus Junior to the Reader', Book 1.

38. See especially Heinzelman, 'Self-interest and the Politics of Composition in Keats's *Isabella*'; see also 'Keats and Politics: A Forum'.

39. Roe, *John Keats*, pp. 226–7.

40. Stillinger, 'Keats and Romance', p. 599.

41. Evan Radcliffe, p. 261.

42. Fraistat, *The Poem and the Book*, pp. 93–140.

43. Stillinger, 'Keats and Romance', p. 603.

44. Carhart-Harris et al., p. 7.

45. Adams, vol. III, p. 423. I am grateful to Gareth Evans for the reference.

46. Thornton, p. 619.

47. See Radden, *Moody Minds Distempered*, pp. 147–65, and Sullivan, *passim*.

48. Kristeva, p. 5.

49. To Reynolds, 25 March, 1818, *LJK*, 1, pp. 262–3.

50. McDowell in 'Grotesque Organicism . . .' argues that the poem is 'part of a self-reflective internal commentary on Keats's own poetics' (p. 23). But her emphasis is different, stressing that the poem is recognised by the poet as not 'organic' and 'neither original nor inspired' but that it 'feeds parasitically off the literary remains of Boccaccio' (p. 22). This seems contentious since the growth of the basil and the decay of the head *are* organic processes. More pertinently here, McDowell refers to 'the apparent recognition that all growth must first have its roots in decay and destruction' (p. 26).

51. Rajan, pp. 129–30.

52. Boccaccio, *The Decameron*.

53. To the George Keatses, 14 February, 1819, *LJK*, 2, pp. 62–3.

54. Gittings, *John Keats: The Living Year*, ch. 8.

55. To Taylor, 17 November, 1819, *LJK*, 2, p. 234.

56. To the George Keatses, 14 February, 1819, *LJK*, 2, p. 62.

57. Contrast, for example, the respective readings by Stillinger in 'The Hoodwinking of Madeline', and Ulmer, pp. 119–24, 133–6.

58. To Bailey, 13 March, 1818, *LJK*, 1, p. 242.

59. Stillinger, *The Hoodwinking of Madeline*, p. 86.

60. Wolfson, 'Keats's "Gordian Complication" of Women', pp. 77–85, 83.

61. Arsenau, 'Madeline, Mermaids and Medusas'.

62. Kübler-Ross, *On Death and Dying*.

63. See Parisot, *Graveyard Poetry*.

64. Woodhouse to Taylor, 19 September, 1819, *LJK*, 2, pp. 162–3.

65. See Gittings, *John Keats: The Living Year*, 'Appendix A', p. 219.

66. See R. S. White, 'Shakespearean Music in Keats's "Ode to a Nightingale"'.

67. Coleridge, 'The Nightingale: A Conversation Poem, April 1798' [orig. publ. in *Lyrical Ballads* (1798)] in *Coleridge: Selected Poems*, ed. John Colmer.

68. To George Keatses, 15–30 April, 1819, *LJK*, 2, p. 89.

69. Matthews, p. 173.

70. 'To Charles Cowden Clarke'.

71. Minahan, p. 173.
72. Evans, 'Poison Wine', pp. 45–6. Goellnicht, pp. 226–7 quotes from Astley Cooper's *The Principles and Practice of Surgery* describing a concussed patient as having 'drunk of the cup of Lethe ... in a state of perfect oblivion'. The image occurs again in 'Ode on Melancholy'.
73. See, for example, Goellnicht, pp. 227–8.
74. Ghosh, *John Keats' Medical Notebook*, pp. 258–9.
75. Noted by Hollander, pp. 90–1.
76. John Jones, p. 167.
77. Jack, pp. 220–1.
78. Eilittä, 'Introduction', in Eilittä and Riccio-Berry, p. ix. In this book see also Klara Franz, 'Externalizing the Picture Frame: Keats's *Negative Capability* and the Uses of Ekphrasis', ch. 2, though this essay does not deal with 'Ode on a Grecian Urn'.
79. See the important discussions of ekphrasis in Keats in Heffernan, *Museum of Words: The Poetics of Ekphrasis from Homer to Ashberry*, Grant F. Scott, *The Sculptured Word*, and Kelley, pp. 170–85.
80. Heffernan, p. 111.
81. Wasserman, *The Finer Tone*, esp. pp. 34–5.
82. Holly, pp. xix–xx.
83. Quoted Holly, p. xxi.
84. Hayden White, 'The Dark Side of Art History'.
85. Greenblatt, *Shakespearean Negotiations: The Circulation of Social Energy in Renaissance England*, p. 1.
86. de Almeida, *Romantic Medicine*, p. 120.
87. It would be futile to supply references to discussions of these lines since they would have to include virtually all editions and critical studies of Keats's odes.
88. Wasserman, p. 13.
89. To the George Keatses, April 30, 1819, *LJK*, 2, pp. 105–6.
90. *King Lear* 1.1.82–3, 85–6.
91. Ulmer, pp. 180–1.
92. Vendler, p. 50.
93. Garrod, pp. 98–9.
94. Bushnell, p. 292.
95. John Jones, pp. 205–6.
96. Stillinger, *The Hoodwinking of Madeline*, pp. 104–5.
97. Ulmer, p. 6, argues for the currency of all these synonyms for 'soul' in Keats's time, while Chandler, p. 7, links the ode more specifically to Keats's comments on 'the vale of Soul-making' in the letter in which the ode was transcribed.
98. Vendler, p. 53.
99. Klibansky et al., p. 153.
100. To Tom Keats, 1 July, 1818, *LJK*, 1, p. 308.
101. To Reynolds, 3 February, 1818, *LJK*, 1, p. 224.
102. Fraistat, *The Poem and the Book*, pp. 127–8.
103. See Robinson, *Unfettering Poetry: The Fancy in British Romanticism* who associates this kind of poetry with Leigh Hunt especially.
104. To George Keatses, January 2, 1819; *LJK*, 2, p. 26.

105. Barnard, 'Keats's "Robin Hood"'.
106. Ibid. p. 184.
107. To the George Keatses, 18 August–1 December 1818, *LJK*, 1, p. 394.
108. To Reynolds, 21 September 1819, *LJK*, 2, p. 167.
109. For example, see McGann, 'Keats and the Historical Method in Literary Criticism', Watkins, *Keats's Poetry and the Politics of the Imagination*, Roe, *John Keats and the Culture of Dissent*, pp. 230–67, Chandler, pp. 426–7. For other recent political readings, see also Paulin, *The Secret Life of Poems: A Poetry Primer* and Turley, Archer and Thomas, 'Keats, "To Autumn", and the New Men of Winchester'.
110. Roe, *John Keats*, pp. 354–5.
111. Hartman, 'Poem and Ideology: A Study of Keats's "To Autumn"'.
112. Turley, 'Objects of Suspicion: Keats, "To Autumn" and the Psychology of Romantic Surveillance'.
113. To Reynolds, 21 September, 1819, *LJK*, 2, p. 167.
114. To Brown, 22 September, 1819, *LJK*, 2, p. 176.
115. Book 1, Memb. III, Subsect. II.
116. To Fanny Brawne, 13 Sept. 1819, *LJK*, 2, p. 160.
117. The phrase 'Let be' occurs in the Second Quarto of Shakespeare's text, and is not included in some modern editions based on the Folio and First Quarto readings.
118. To Bailey, 22 November, 1817, *LJK*, 1, p. 186.
119. To George and Tom, Keats 21–7, 1817, *LJK*, 1, p. 192.
120. Bate, *John Keats*, p. 581.
121. Jack, p. 235.
122. Plumly, p. 304.
123. Ulmer, pp. 202–3.
124. To Reynolds, 22 November, 1817, *LJK*, 1, p. 189.
125. Stevens, *The Collected Poems of Wallace Stevens*.
126. R. S. White, *John Keats: A Literary Life*, pp. 201–6
127. To George and Tom Keats, 14(?) February, 1818, *LJK*, 1, p. 227. Hazlitt's lecture appears in *Lectures on the English Poets*, Lecture V.
128. Thomson, pp. 162–3.
129. Turley, *Keats's Places*, p. 239.
130. To Reynolds, 21 September, 1819, *LJK*, 2, p. 167.
131. Jack, pp. 235–8.
132. Henderson, p. 235.
133. To George Keatses April, 21 1819, *LJK*, 2, p. 101.
134. Fry, p. 217.
135. Ghosh, *John Keats' Medical Notebook*, p. 160.
136. Pladek, p. 165.
137. Klibansky et al., p. 238.
138. Keats, *The Complete Poems* ed. Miriam Allott, p. 539.
139. As a rather irrelevant digression, in a letter to Fanny Brawne in May 1820 Keats wrote, 'I cannot brook the wolfsbane of fashion, flattery and tattle'. It seems in context to denote a dangerous social poison.
140. de Almeida, *Romantic Medicine*, p. 171.
141. Evans, 'Poison Wine', p. 53. For more detail on the 'poison fruits' see de Almeida, *Romantic Medicine*, pp. 168–74.

142. Ghosh traces the references in Culpepper as well; *John Keats' Medical Notebook*, pp. 260–1.
143. Henderson, p. 240.
144. To Reynolds, 22 November, 1817 *LJK*, 1, p. 189.
145. de Almeida, *Romantic Medicine*, p. 172.
146. Radden, *Melancholy: From Aristotle to Kristeva*, p. 220.
147. To Haydon, 23 January, 1818, *LJK*, 1, p. 207.
148. Sperry, p. 188.
149. Fraistat, *The Poem and the Book*, p. 214, fn. 49.
150. Ziegenhagen, p. 292.
151. Muir, p. 120ff.
152. To the George Keatses, 18 December, 1818, *LJK*, 2, p. 12.
153. To Sarah Jeffrey, 31 May 1819, *LJK*, 2, p. 113.
154. Sperry, p. 294.
155. To Bailey, 8 October, 1817, *LJK*, 1, pp. 169–70.

Bibliography

'Aesculapius', *Oracular Communications, addressed to Students of the Medical Profession,* London: E. Cox and Son, 1816.

'Aesculapius', *The Hospital Pupil's Guide, being Oracular Communications, addressed to Students of the Medical Profession,* London: E. Cox and Son, 1818.

Adams, Francis (trans.), *The Seven Books of Paulus AEginata Translated from the Greek,* 3 vols, London: The Sydenham Society, 1847.

Almeida, Hermione de, *Romantic Medicine and John Keats,* New York and Oxford: Oxford University Press, 1991.

Arikha, Nola, *Passions and Tempers: A History of the Humours,* New York: HarperCollins, 2007.

Arseneau, Mary, 'Madeline, Mermaids, and Medusas in "The Eve of St Agnes"', *Papers on Language and Literature*; 33 (Summer, 1997), 227–42.

Bamborough, J. B., 'Introduction', *Robert Burton: The Anatomy of Melancholy,* ed. Thomas C. Faulkner et al., Oxford: Clarendon Press, 1989–1992, vol. 1, xiii–xxxvii.

Bari, Shahidha, *Keats and Philosophy: The Life of Sensations,* London: Routledge, 2012.

Barnard, John, 'Keats's "Robin Hood", John Hamilton Reynolds, and the "Old Poets"', *Proceedings of the British Academy,* 75 (1989), 181–200.

Barnard, John, 'First Fruits or "First Blights": A New Account of the Publishing History of Keats's Poems' (1817), *Romanticism,* 12 (2006), 71–93.

Barnard, John, '"The busy time": Keats's duties at Guy's Hospital from Autumn 1816 to March 1817', *Romanticism,* 13 (2007), 199–218.

Barthes, Roland, *S|Z,* trans. Richard Miller, London: Jonathan Cape, 1975.

Barthes, Roland, *Image-Music-Text.* Essays collected and trans. by Stephen Heath, London: Fontana Press, 1977.

Bate, W. J., *John Keats,* Cambridge, MA: Harvard University Press, 1964.

Bate, W. J., *Negative Capability: The Intuitive Approach in Keats,* Cambridge, MA: Harvard University Press, 1939.

Bate, W. J., *Samuel Johnson,* New York: Harcourt, Brace, Jovanovich, 1977.

Bennett, Andrew, *Keats, Narrative and Audience: The Posthumous Life of Writing,* Cambridge: Cambridge University Press, 1994.

Bernard, J. F., *Shakespearean Melancholy: Philosophy, Form, and the Transformation of Comedy,* Edinburgh: Edinburgh University Press, 2018.

Bion, Wilfred, *Attention and Interpretation. A Scientific Approach to Insight in Psycho-Analysis and Groups,* London: Tavistock, 1970, reprinted London: Karnac Books, 1984.

Blunden, Edmund, *John Keats,* London: Longmans and the British Council, 1959.

Blunden, Edmund, *Keats's Publisher: A Memoir of John Taylor (1781–1864),* London: Jonathan Cape, 1936.

Blunden, Edmund, *London Mercury,* 4 (1921).

Boccaccio, Giovanni, *The Decameron Containing An hundred pleasant Novels. Wittily discoursed, betweene seaven Honourable Ladies, and three Noble Gentlemen,* London: Isaac Jaggard, 1620.

Boswell, James, *Boswell's Life of Johnson,* ed. Sir Sydney Roberts, 2 vols, London: J. M. Dent & Sons, 1960.

Boyce, Niall and Gareth Evans, 'The art of medicine: Nothing but flowers', *The Lancet,* vol. 378 (2011), Issue 9802, 1541–2.

Brand, D. P., *Italy and the English Romantics: The Italianate Fashion in Nineteenth Century Literature,* Cambridge: Cambridge University Press, 1957.

Brown, Charles Armitage, *Life of John Keats* [written 1836], ed. Dorothy Hyde Bodurtha and Willard B. Pope, London: Oxford University Press, 1937.

Bubenik, Andrea (ed.), *Five Centuries of Melancholia,* Brisbane: University of Queensland Art Gallery, 2014.

Burch, Druin, 'Astley Paston Cooper (1786–1841): Anatomist, Radical, Surgeon', *The James Lindley Library Bulletin* (2009) <http://www.james lindlibrary.org/articles/astley-paston-cooper-1768-1841-anatomist-radical-and-surgeon/> (last accessed 20 March 2020).

Burch, Druin, 'The Beauty of Bodysnatching' *John Keats and the Medical Imagination,* ed. Nicholas Roe, London: Palgrave, 2017, 43–56.

Burton, Robert ('Democritus Junior'), *The Anatomy of Melancholy,* London and Oxford: sundry editions, 1621–1676.

Burton, Robert, *The Anatomy of Melancholy,* 2 vols, 11th edn, London: J. Walker et al., 1813.

Burton, Robert, *The Anatomy of Melancholy,* 2 vols, 12th edn, London: J. Cuthell et al., 1821. Vol. 2 available as digital facsimile at <https://archive.org/stream/b29328433_0002?ref=ol#page/n6/mode/2up> (last accessed 20 March 2020).

Burton, Robert, *The Anatomy of Melancholy,* ed. Holbrook Jackson, London: J. M. Dent Everyman Library, 1932.

Burton, Robert, *Robert Burton: The Anatomy of Melancholy,* ed. Thomas C. Faulkner et al., Oxford: Clarendon Press, vols 1–3, 1989–1992.

Burton, Robert, 'Marginalia in Burton's *The Art of Melancholy,* Royal College of Physicians of Edinburgh <http://www.rcpe.ac.uk/heritage/marginalia-burt ons-anatomy-melancholy-1821> (last accessed 20 March 2020).

Bushnell, Nelson Sherwin, 'Notes on Professor Garrod's *Keats', Modern Language Notes,* 5 (1929), 287–96.

Campbell, Laura E., 'Unnecessary Compromise: Publisher Changes to "Ode to Psyche"', *English Language Notes,* 33 (1995), 53–8.

Campbell, R., *The London Tradesman,* London: 1747. Facsimile available at

<https://archive.org/details/TheLondonTradesman/page/n7/mode/2up> (last accessed 20 March 2020).

Carhart-Harris, Robin L. et al., 'Mourning and melancholia revisited: correspondences between principles of Freudian metapsychology and empirical findings in neuropsychiatry', *Annals of General Psychiatry*, 7 (2008), 1–23.

Chambers, Jane, '"For love's sake": Lamia and Burton's Melancholy', *Studies in English Literature, 1500–1900*, 2 (1982), 583–600.

Chandler, James, *England in 1819: The Politics of Literary Culture and the Case of Romantic Historicism*, Chicago: The University of Chicago Press, 1978.

Chilcott, Tim, *A Publisher and his Circle: The Life and Work of John Taylor, Keats's Publisher*, London: Routledge & Kegan Paul, 1972.

Clarke, Charles Cowden, ' Recollections of Keats by An Old School-Fellow', *Atlantic Monthly* 7 (Jan 1861), 86–100.

Clucas, Tom, 'Medicalized Sensibility: Keats and *The Florence Miscellany*', *Keats-Shelley Review* 25 (2011), 122–36.

Coleridge, S. T., *Coleridge: Selected Poems*, ed. John Colmer, Oxford: Oxford University Press, 1965.

Cooper, Astley, 'The Hunterian Oration on Astley Cooper and Hunterian Principles', *The Lancet*, Feb. 19 (1921).

Cooper, Astley, *John Keats's Anatomical and Physiological Note Book*, ed. Maurice Buxton Forman, New York: Haskell House Publishers, 1970.

Cornish, Sally, 'Negative Capability and Social Work: Insights from Keats, Bion and Business', *Journal of Social Work Practice*, 25 (2011), 135–46.

Cox, Jeffrey N., '*Lamia, Isabella*, and *The Eve of St Agnes*: Eros and "Romance"', in Susan J. Wolfson (ed.), *The Cambridge Companion to Keats*, Cambridge: Cambridge University Press, 2001, 53–68.

Cox, Jeffrey N. (ed.), *Keats's Poetry and Prose*, New York: W. W. Norton, 2009.

Curran, Stuart, *Poetic Form and British Romanticism*, New York, Oxford: Oxford University Press, 1986.

Davies, Damian Walford, 'Keats's Killing Breath: Paradigms of a Pathology', in Nicholas Roe (ed.), *John Keats and the Medical Imagination*, London: Palgrave Macmillan, 2017, 207–42.

Dixon, Laurinda S., 'Mind over Madness: The Development of the Topos of the Melancholic Artist', in Andrew Lynch and Susan Broomhall (eds), *The Routledge History of Emotions in Europe, 1100–1700*, London: 2019, 435–50.

Dodsworth, Martin, 'Textual Introduction: Publishing History: The Growth of *The Anatomy of Melancholy*', in Thomas C. Faulkner, Nicolas K. Kiessling and Rhonda L. Blair (eds), *Robert Burton: The Anatomy of Melancholy*, Oxford: Clarendon Press, 1989.

Dunbar, Georgia S., 'The Significance of the Humor in "Lamia"', *Keats-Shelley Journal*, 8 (1959), 17–26.

Eilittä, Leina H. and Catherine Riccio-Berry, *Afterlives of Romantic Intermediality: The Interactions of Visual, Aural, and Verbal Frontiers*, London: Lexington Books, 2016.

Eliot, T. S., 'Hamlet and his Problems', *The Sacred Wood*, London: Faber and Faber, 1921.

Enderwitz, Anne, *Modernist Melancholia: Freud, Conrad and Ford*, London: Palgrave Macmillan, 2015.

Evans, Gareth, 'Poison Wine – John Keats and the Botanic Pharmacy', *Keats-Shelley Review*, 16 (2002), 31–55.

Evans, Gareth, 'Nice Ink, Keats. The medical student and his botanical literary doodle', Dove Cottage and the Wordsworth Museum, January 2019 <https://wordsworth.org.uk/blog/2019/01/21/nice-ink-keats/> (last accessed 20 March 2020).

Falkes, Cassandra, 'Negatively Capable Reading' in Brian Rejack and Michael Theune (eds), *Keats's Negative Capability: New Origins and Afterlives*, Liverpool: Liverpool University Press, 2019, 47–59.

Ferriar, John M. D., *Illustrations of Sterne with Other Essays and Verses*, London: Cadell and Davies, 1798.

Fitzpatrick, Joan, *Food in Shakespeare: Early Modern Dietaries and the Plays*, London: Routledge, 2016.

Fraistat, Neil, *The Poem and the Book: Interpreting Collections of Romantic Poetry*, Chapel Hill: University of North Carolina, 1985.

Fraistat, Neil (ed.), *Poems in Their Place: The Intertextuality and Order of Poetic Collections*, Chapel Hill: University of North Carolina, 1986.

French, R. and P. Simpson, "Negative Capability and the Capacity to Think in the Present Moment" *Leadership*, 2 (2006): 245–55.

Freud, Sigmund, *The Standard Edition of the Complete Psychological Works of Sigmund Freud*, gen. ed. James Strachey, 24 vols, London: Hogarth Press, 1956–74.

Fry, Paul H., 'History, Existence, and "To Autumn"', *Studies in Romanticism* 25 (1986), 211–19.

Gamer, Michael, *Romanticism, Self-Canonization, and the Business of Poetry*, Cambridge: Cambridge University Press, 2017.

Garrod, H. W., *Keats*, Oxford: Oxford University Press, 1926.

Ghosh, Hrileena, 'John Keats's "Guy's Hospital" Poetry', in Nicholas Roe (ed.), *John Keats and the Medical Imagination*, London: Palgrave, 2017, 1–20.

Ghosh, Hrileena, 'Keats at Guy's Hospital: Moments, Meetings, Choices, and Poems' in Richard Marggraf Turley (ed.), *Keats's Places*, London: Palgrave, 2018, 31–52.

Ghosh, Hrileena, *John Keats' Medical Notebook: Text, Context and Poems*, Liverpool: Liverpool University Press, 2020.

Gibson, Andrew, 'Oublier Baudrillard: Melancholy of the Year 2000', *New Formations* 50 (2003), 123–41.

Gill, Stephen, *Wordsworth's Revisitings*, Oxford: Oxford University Press, 2011.

Gittings, Robert, *John Keats: The Living Year*, London: Heinemann, 1954.

Gittings, Robert, *John Keats*, London: Heinemann, 1968.

Gittings, Robert, *The Odes of Keats and their Earliest Known Manuscripts*, Kent, Ohio: Kent State University Press, 1970.

Goellnicht, Donald C., *The Poet-Physician: Keats and Medical Science*, Pittsburgh: University of Pittsburgh Press, 1984.

Gowland, Angus, 'Melancholy, Imagination, and Dreaming in Renaissance Learning' in Yasmin Haskell (ed.), *Diseases of the Imagination and Imaginary*

Disease in the Early Modern Period, Turnhout, Belgium: Brepols, 2011, 54–102, 56.

Gowland, Angus, 'Rhetorical Structure and Function in *The Anatomy of Melancholy*', *Rhetorica*, 19 (2001), 1–48.

Gowland, Angus, 'The Problem of Early Modern Melancholy', *Past and Present*, 191 (2006), 77–120.

Gowland, Angus, *The Worlds of Renaissance Melancholy: Robert Burton in Context*, Cambridge: Cambridge University Press, 2006.

Greenblatt, Stephen, *Renaissance Self-Fashioning: From More to Shakespeare*, Chicago: Chicago University Press, 1980.

Greenblatt, Stephen, *Shakespearean Negotiations: The Circulation of Social Energy in Renaissance England*, Oxford: Clarendon Press, 1988, 1.

Greenblatt, Stephen (ed.), *Norton Anthology of English Literature: The Restoration and the Eighteenth Century*, 9th edn, New York: W. W. Norton, 2012.

Greenblatt, Stephen, 'King Lear, a difficult play, not helped by sloppy analysis', *Financial Review*, Feb. 14, 2017; repr. From *New York Review of Books*.

Grinnell, George C., *The Age of Hypochondria: Interpreting Romantic Health and Illness*, London: Palgrave Macmillan, 2010.

Haley, Bruce, *Living Forms: Romantics and the Monumental Figure*, Albany, NY: State University of New York Press, 2003.

Hall, John, *John Hall and his Patients: The Medical Practice of Shakespeare's Son-in-Law*, ed. Joan Lane, Stratford Upon Avon: The Shakespeare Birthplace Trust, 2001.

Harlan, David, 'Intellectual History and the Return of Literature', *The American Historical Review*, 94 (1989), 581–609.

Hartman, Geoffrey, 'Poem and Ideology: A Study of Keats's "To Autumn"', *The Fate of Reading*, Chicago: The University of Chicago Press, 1975, 124–46.

Haskell, Yasmin (ed.), *Diseases of the Imagination and Imaginary Disease in the Early Modern Period*, Turnhout, Belgium: Brepols, 2011.

Haworth, Helen, 'Keats's Copy of Lamb's *Specimens of English Dramatic Poets*', *Bulletin of the New York Public Library*, 74 (1970), 419–27.

Hay, Daisy, 'Elizabeth Kent's Collaborators', *Romanticism*, 14 (2008), 272–80.

Haydon, Benjamin, *The Diary of Benjamin Haydon*, ed. W. B. Pope, Cambridge MA: Harvard University Press, 1960.

Hazlitt, William, *Lectures on the English Poets*, London: Taylor and Hessey, 1818.

Hazlitt, William, 'On Gusto', First published in *The Examiner*, 26 May, 1816, repr. *The Round Table*, London: Sampson Low, Son, & Marston, 1869.

Hazlitt, William, *The Complete Works of William Hazlitt*, ed. P. P. Howe, 21 vols, London and Toronto: J. M. Dent, 1930–4.

Heffernan, James A., *Museum of Words: The Poetics of Ekphrasis from Homer to Ashberry*, Chicago: The University of Chicago Press, 1993.

Heinzelman, Kurt, 'Self-interest and the Politics of Composition in Keats's *Isabella*', *English Literary History*, 55 (1998), 159–93.

Henderson, Andrea, 'Mastery and Melancholy in Suburbia', *The Eighteenth Century*, 50 (2009), 221–44.

Herford, Oliver, 'Joseph Severn: On Likeness and Life-Writing', *The Cambridge Quarterly*, 42 (2013), 318–41.

Hersey, George L., *Alfonso II and the artistic renewal of Naples, 1485–1495*, New Haven: Yale University Press, 1969.

Hessell, Nikki, 'John Keats, the Botanist's Companion', in Nicholas Roe (ed.), *John Keats and the Medical Imagination*, London: Palgrave Macmillan, 2017, 91–108.

Hoeveler, Diane, 'Decapitating Romance: Class, Fetish, and Ideology in Keats's *Isabella*', *Nineteenth-Century Literature*, 49 (1994), 321–38.

Holland, Norman, *5 Readers Reading*, New Haven: Yale University Press, 1975.

Hollander, John, *The Figure of Echo: A Mode of Allusion in Milton and After*, Berkeley: University of California Press, 1981.

Holloway, S. W. F., 'The Apothecaries' Act, 1815: A Reinterpretation. Part 1. The Origins of the Act', *Medical History*, 10.2 (1966), 107–29.

Holloway, S. W. F., 'The Apothecaries' Act, 1815: A Reinterpretation. Part 2. The Consequences of the Act', *Medical History*, 10.3 (1966), 221–36.

Holly, Michael Ann, *The Melancholy Art*, Princeton: Princeton University Press, 2013.

Homans, Margaret, 'Keats Reading Women, Women Reading Keats'. *Studies in Romanticism*, 29 (1990), 341–70.

Hughes, William, David Punter and Andrew Smith (eds), *The Encyclopedia of the Gothic*, 2 vols, Oxford: Wiley-Blackwell, 2013.

Iser, Wolfgang, *The Act of Reading: A Theory of Aesthetic Response*, London: Routledge & Kegan Paul, 1978.

Jack, Ian, *Keats and the Mirror of Art*, Oxford: Clarendon Press, 1965.

Jackson, Stanley W., *Melancholia and Depression: From Hippocratic Times to Modern Times*, New Haven and London: Yale University Press, 1986.

Jauss, Hans Robert, *Toward an Aesthetic of Reception*, trans. Timothy Bahti, Brighton: Harvester Press, 1982.

Jones, Chris, *Radical Sensibility: Literature and Ideas in the 1790s*, London: Routledge, 1993.

Jones, John, *John Keats's Dream of Truth*, London: Chatto and Windus, 1969.

'Keats and Politics: A Forum', *Studies in Romanticism*, 25.2 (Summer 1986).

Keats, John, *Keats: Poems Published in 1820*, ed. M. Robertson, Oxford: Oxford University Press, 1909.

Keats, John, *The Complete Works of John Keats*, ed. H. Buxton Forman, rev. M. Buxton Forman, 8 vols, Hampstead Edition, New York: Charles Scribner's Sons, 1938.

Keats, John, *The Keats Circle*, ed. Hyder Rollins, 2 vols, Cambridge, MA: Harvard University Press, 1948.

Keats, John, *The Keats Circle: Letters and Papers and More Letters and Poems of the Keats Circle*, 2nd edn, ed. Hyder E. Rollins, 2 vols, Cambridge, MA: Harvard University Press, 1965.

Keats, John, *The Complete Poems*, ed. Miriam Allott, London: Longman, 1970.

Keats, John, *John Keats's Anatomical and Physiological Note Book*, ed. Maurice Buxton Forman [1934], New York: Haskell House Publishers Ltd, 1970.

Keats, John. *The Complete Poems*, Penguin English Poets, 3rd rev. edn, ed. John Barnard, Harmondsworth: Penguin Books, 1977.

Keats, John, *The Poems of John Keats*, ed. Jack Stillinger, London: Heinemann, 1978.

Keats, John, *Lamia, Isabella, The Eve of St Agnes and Other Poems, with 'Note on the Text' by Michael Schmidt*. Penguin Poetry First Edition, London: Penguin Books, 1999.

Keats, John, *Lamia, Isabella, The Eve of St Agnes 1820*. Facsimile, Otley, Washington, DC: Woodstock Books, 2001.

Keats, John, *The Letters of John Keats 1814–1821*, ed. Hyder Edward Rollins, 2 vols, Cambridge, MA: Harvard University Press, 2002.

Keats, John, *John Keats: 21st-Century Oxford Authors*, ed. John Barnard, Oxford: Oxford University Press, 2017.

Keats, John, *John Keats: Selected Letters*, ed. John Barnard, London: Penguin Classics, 2014.

Kelley, Theresa M., 'Keats and Ekphrasis', in Susan J. Wolfson (ed.), *The Cambridge Companion to Keats*, Cambridge: Cambridge University Press, 2001, 170–85.

Kent, Elizabeth, *Flora Domestica, or The Portable Flower-Garden*, London: Taylor and Hessey, 1821. <https://archive.org/details/floradomesticaor00ken trich/page/n5> (last accessed 20 March 2020).

Keymer, Thomas, *Sterne, the Moderns, and the Novel*, Oxford: Oxford University Press, 2002, 153–4.

Klibansky, Raymond, Erwin Panofsky and Fritz Saxl, *Saturn and Melancholy: Studies in the History of Natural Philosophy, Religion and Art*, London, 1964, reprint Nendeln Liechenstcin, 1979.

Kristeva, Julia, 'On the Melancholic Imaginary', *New Formations*, 3 (1987), 5–17.

Kübler-Ross, Elisabeth, *On Death and Dying*, London: Routledge, 1969.

Lamb, Charles and Mary, *Works of Charles and Mary Lamb*, vols V–VI, in E. V. Lucas (ed.), *Letters*, London: Methuen, 1913.

Lamb, Charles, *Specimens of English Dramatic Poets, Who Lived About the Time of Shakespeare*, London: Longman, Hurst, Rees, and Orme, 1808.

Lane, Joan, 'The role of apprenticeship in eighteenth-century medical education in England', in W. F. Byrnum and Roy Porter (eds), *William Hunter and the Eighteenth-Century Medical World*, Cambridge: Cambridge University Press, 2002, 57–103.

Lau, Beth, *Keats's Paradise Lost*, Gainesville: University Press of Florida, 1998.

Lau, Beth, 'John Keats' in Adrian Poole (ed.), *Lamb, Hazlitt, Keats: Great Shakespeareans*, London: Continuum, 2010, vol. IV, 109–59.

Lau, Beth, 'Analyzing Keats's Library by Genre', *Keats-Shelley Journal*, 65 (2016), 126–51.

Lawrence, D. H., *The Complete Poems of D. H. Lawrence*, ed. Vivian de Sola Pinto and Warren Roberts, London: Heinemann, 1964.

Lowell, Amy, *John Keats*, 2 vols, Boston: Houghton Mifflin, 1925.

Lowes, John Livingston, 'The lovers maladye of hereos', *Modern Philology*, 11 (1914), 491–546.

Lynch, Andrew and Susan Broomhall (eds), *The Routledge History of Emotions in Europe, 1100–1700*, London: Routledge, 2019.

Mark, Raymond, *Marked by melancholy: The character of the pensive text in*

Gray and Keats, New York University, ProQuest Dissertations Publishing, 2005.

Martz, Louis L., 'George Herbert: The Unity of *The Temple*', *The Poetry of Meditation*, New Haven: Yale University Press, 1954.

Matthews, G. M., *Keats: The Critical Heritage*, London: Routledge and Kegan Paul, 1971.

McDowell, Stacey, 'Grotesque organicism in Keats's *Isabella; or, The Pot of Basil*', *The Keats- Shelley Review*, 24 (2013), 22–8.

McGann, Jerome, 'Keats and the Historical Method in Literary Criticism', *Modern Language Notes*, 94 (1979).

McQuillan, Martin, 'Introduction: There Is No Such Thing as Reader-Response Theory', in Julian Wolfreys (ed.), *Literary Theories: A Reader and A Guide*, Edinburgh: Edinburgh University Press, 1999, 139–48, 139.

Mee, Jon, '"Reciprocal Expressions of Kindness": Robert Merry, Della Cruscanism and the Limits of Sociability', in Gillian Russell and Clara Tuite, *Romantic Sociability: Social Networks and Literary Culture in Britain, 1770–1840*, Cambridge: Cambridge University Press, 2002, 104–22.

Mellor, Anne, 'Keats and the Complexities of Gender', in *The Cambridge Companion to Keats*, Susan Wolfson (ed.), Cambridge: Cambridge University Press, 2001, 214–29.

Middeke, Martin and Christina Wald (eds), *The Literature of Melancholia: Early Modern to Postmodern*, London: Palgrave Macmillan, 2011.

Milton, John, *Poems Upon Several Occasions*, ed. Thomas Warton, London: 1785.

Milton, John, *Milton's Sonnets*, ed. E. A. J. Honigmann, London: Macmillan, 1966.

Minahan, John A., *Word Like a Bell: John Keats, Music and the Romantic Poet*, Kent, OH: Kent State University Press, 1992.

Moore, W., *The Knife Man: Blood, Body-Snatching and the Birth of Modern Surgery*, London: Bantam Books, 2005.

Motion, Andrew, *John Keats*, London: Faber and Faber, 1997.

Muir, Kenneth (ed.), *John Keats: A Reassessment*, Liverpool: Liverpool University Press, 1958.

Murray, John, *A System of Materia Medica and Pharmacy*, 2 vols, Edinburgh: W. Laing, J. Anderson, J. Bathgate, Brown & Crombie, and A. Black, 1810.

New, Melvyn, *Tristram Shandy: A Book for Free Spirits*, New York: Twayne Publishers, 1994.

Nowotny, Helga, *The Cunning of Uncertainty*, London: Polity, 2017.

O'Brien, Sean, 'An Ode to John Keats'. Radio podcast, broadcast 8 January 2019. <https://www.bbc.co.uk/sounds/play/m0001xwj> (last accessed 20 March 2020).

O'Halloran, Meiko, 'Reawakening Lycidas: Keats, Milton, and the Epic', *Review of English Studies*, May 2019 eprint.

O'Neill, Michael, *John Keats in Context*, Cambridge: Cambridge University Press, 2017.

Ou, Li, *Keats and Negative Capability*, London: Continuum, 2009.

Owings, Frank, *The Keats Library: A Descriptive Catalogue*, London: Keats-Shelley Memorial Association, 1978.

Parisot, Eric, *Graveyard Poetry: Religion, Aesthetics and the Mid-Eighteenth-Century Poetic Condition*, Farnham: Ashgate, 2013.

Parnell, Rev. Thomas, *The Poetical Works of Thomas Parnell, The Aldine Edition of the British Poets*, London: Bell and Daldy, 1866, 93.

Patterson, Charles I., *The Daemonic in the Poetry of John Keats*, Urbana: University of Illinois Press, 1970.

Paulin, Tom, *The Secret Life of Poems: A Poetry Primer*, London: Faber and Faber, 2011.

Pladek, Brittany, *The Poetics of Palliation: Romantic Literary Therapy*, Liverpool: Liverpool University Press, 2019.

Plumly, Stanley, *Posthumous Keats: A Personal Biography*, New York: W. W. Norton, 2008.

Porter, Roy, 'The Patient's View: Doing Medical History from Below', *Theory and Society*, 14 (1985), 175–98, 193.

Porter, Roy, *Blood and Guts: A Short History of Medicine*, London: Penguin, 2002.

Porter, Roy, *Flesh in the Age of Reason*, New York: Allen Lane, 2004.

Radcliffe, Ann, *The Mysteries of Udolpho*, 4 vols, London: G. G and J. Robinson, 1794.

Radcliffe, Evan, 'Keats, Ideals, and *Isabella*', *Modern Language Quarterly*, 47 (1986).

Radden, Jennifer, *The Nature of Melancholy from Aristotle to Kristeva*, New York: Oxford University Press, 2000.

Radden, Jennifer, *Moody Minds Distempered: Essays on Melancholy and Depression*, New York: Oxford University Press, 2009.

Rajan, Tilottama, *Dark Interpreter: The Discourse of Romanticism*, Ithaca: Cornell University Press, 1980.

Read, Herbert, *The Contrary Experience*, London: Faber & Faber, 1963.

Rejack, Brian and Michael Theune (eds), *Keats's Negative Capability: New Origins and Afterlives*, Liverpool: Liverpool University Press, 2019.

Reyes, Xavier Aldana (ed.), *Horror: A Literary History*, London: The British Library, 2016.

Reynolds, John Hamilton, *The Letters of John Hamilton Reynolds*, ed. Leonidas M. Jones, Lincoln: University of Nebraska Press, 1973.

Ricks, Christopher, *Keats and Embarrassment*, Oxford: Oxford University Press, 1974.

Rivlin J. J., 'Getting a medical qualification in England in the nineteenth century', *Medical Historian*, 9 (1997): 56–63.

Robinson, Jeffrey C., *Unfettering Poetry: The Fancy in British Romanticism*, London: Palgrave Macmillan, 2006.

Roe, Nicholas, *John Keats and the Culture of Dissent*, Oxford: Clarendon Press, 1997.

Roe, Nicholas, 'Undefinitive Keats', in Ashley Chantler, Michael Davies and Philip Shaw (eds), *Literature and Authenticity: Essays in Honour of Vincent Newey*, Farnham: Ashgate, 2011.

Roe, Nicholas, *John Keats: A New Life*, New Haven: Yale University Press, 2012.

Roe, Nicholas (ed.), *John Keats and the Medical Imagination*, London: Palgrave, 2017.

Ruston, Sharon, 'John Keats, Poet-Physician', *Discovering Literature: Romantics and Victorians*, British Library <https://www.bl.uk/romantics-and-victorians/articles/john-keats-poet-physician> (last accessed 20 March 2020).

Schiesari, Julian, *The Gendering of Melancholia: Feminism, Psychoanalysis, and the Symbolics of Loss in Renaissance Literature*, Ithaca: Cornell University Press, 1992.

Schor, Naomi, *One Hundred Years of Melancholy*, Oxford: Clarendon Press, 1996.

Schulkins, Rachel, *Keats, Modesty and Masturbation*, London: Routledge, 2014.

Scott, Grant F., 'Keats's American Ode' in Richard Marggraf Turley (ed.), *Keats's Places*, London: Palgrave, 2018, 205–24.

Scott, Grant F., *The Sculptured Word: Keats, Ekphrasis and the Visual Arts*, Hanover: University Press of New England, 1994.

Shakespeare, William, *The Arden Shakespeare Complete Works*, ed. Richard Proudfoot, Ann Thompson and David Scott Kastan, London: The Arden Shakespeare, 1998.

Sigler, David, 'Negative Capability in Psychoanalysis: Keats and Retroactive Judgment in Bion, Freud, Lacan and Milner', in Brian Rejack and Michael Theune (eds), *Keats's Negative Capability: New Origins and Afterlives*, Liverpool: Liverpool University Press, 2019, 216–31.

Sinson, Janice C., *John Keats and the Anatomy of Melancholy*, London: Keats-Shelley Memorial Association, 1971.

Smith, Hillas, *Keats and Medicine*, Newport, Isle of Wight: Cross Publishing, 1995.

Spenser, Edmund, *Poetical Works*, ed. J. C. Smith and E. de Selincourt, Oxford: Oxford University Press, 1912.

Sperry, Stuart, *Keats the Poet*, Princeton: Princeton University Press, 1973.

Spurgeon, Caroline, *Keats's Shakespeare: A Descriptive Study*, Oxford: Oxford University Press, 2nd edn, 1929.

Stevens, Wallace, *The Collected Poems of Wallace Stevens*, New York: Knopf, 1954.

Stillinger, Jack, 'Keats and Romance', *Studies in English Literature*, 8 (1968), 593–605.

Stillinger, Jack, 'The Order of Poems in Keats's First Volume', in *The Hoodwinking of Madeline and Other Essays on Keats's Poems*, Urbana: University of Illinois Press, 1971, 1–13.

Stillinger, Jack, *The Texts of Keats's Poems*, Cambridge, MA: Harvard University Press, 1974.

Stillinger, Jack, 'Review'. *Modern Philology*, 84 (May, 1987), 436–7.

Stillinger, Jack, 'Keats's Extempore Effusions: Questions of Intentionality', in Robert Brinkley and Keith Hanley (eds), *Romantic Revisions*, Cambridge: Cambridge University Press, 1992, 307–20.

Stillinger, Jack, *Reading the Eve of St Agnes: The Multiples of Complex Literary Transaction*, New York: Oxford University Press, 1999.

Stockwell, Peter, *Texture: A Cognitive Aesthetics of Reading*, Edinburgh: Edinburgh University Press, 2009.

Sullivan, Erin, *Beyond Melancholy: Sadness and Selfhood in Renaissance England*, Oxford: Oxford University Press, 2016.

Thomson, James, *Poetical Works*, ed. J. Logie Robertson, London: Oxford University Press, 1908.

Thornton, Robert John, *A Family Herbal or Familiar Account of the Medical Properties of British and Foreign Plants*, 2nd edn, London: B. & R. Crosby & Co., 1814.

Tompkins, Jane P. (ed.), *Reader-Response Criticism: From Formalism to Post-Structuralism*, Baltimore: Johns Hopkins University, 1980.

Turley, Richard Marggraf, *Bright Stars: John Keats, Barry Cornwall, and Romantic Literary Culture*, Liverpool: Liverpool University Press, 2009.

Turley, Richard Marggraf, 'Objects of Suspicion: Keats, "To Autumn" and the Psychology of Romantic Surveillance', *John Keats and the Medical Imagination*, London: Palgrave, 2017, 173–205.

Turley, Richard Marggraf, *Keats's Places*, London: Palgrave, 2018.

Turley, Richard Marggraf, Jayne Elizabeth Archer and Howard Thomas (eds), 'Keats, "To Autumn", and the New Men of Winchester', *Review of English Studies*, 63 (2012), 797–817.

Tuve, Rosamund, *A Reading of George Herbert*, London: Faber, 1952.

Ulmer, William A., *John Keats: Reimagining History*, London: Palgrave Macmillan, 2017.

Vendler, Helen, *The Odes of John Keats*, Cambridge, MA: The Belknap Press of Harvard University Press, 1983.

Voller, Diana, 'Negative Capability: The psychotherapist's X-factor?', in *Existential Analysis*, 22 (2011), 344–55; reprinted in Manu Bazzanu and Julie Webb (eds), *Therapy and the Counter-tradition: The Edge of Philosophy*, London: Routledge, 2016, ch. 3.

Voller, Diana, 'Negative Capability', in *Contemporary Psychotherapy*, 2 (2010). <http://www.contemporarypsychotherapy.org/vol-2-no-2/negative-capabili ty/> (last accessed 20 March 2020).

Ward, Aileen, *John Keats: The Making of a Poet*, New York: Viking Press, 1963.

Warton, Thomas, *The Pleasures of Melancholy: A Poem*, London: 1747.

Warton, Thomas, *Milton: Poems Upon Several Occasions*, London: 1785.

Wasserman, Earl, *The Finer Tone: Keats' Major Poems*, Baltimore: Johns Hopkins University Press, 1953.

Watkins, Daniel P., *Keats's Poetry and the Politics of the Imagination*, Rutherford, NJ: Fairleigh Dickinson University Press, 1989.

Whale, John, *John Keats: Critical Issues*, London: Palgrave Macmillan, 2005.

White, Hayden, 'The Dark Side of Art History', *The Art Bulletin*, 89 (2007), 21–6.

White, R. S., 'Shakespearean Music in Keats's "Ode to a Nightingale"', *English*, 30 (1981), 217–29.

White, R. S., *Keats as a Reader of Shakespeare*, London: Athlone Press, 1987; republ. London: Bloomsbury, 2016.

White, R. S., 'Like Aesculapius of Old': Keats's Medical Training', *Keats-Shelley Review*, 12 (1998), 15–49.

White, R. S., 'Keats and the Crisis of Medicine in 1815', *Keats-Shelley Review*, 13 (1999) 58–75.

White, R. S., *Natural Rights and the Birth of Romanticism in the 1790s*, London: Palgrave, 2005.

White, R. S., *John Keats: A Literary Life*, London: Palgrave, 2010, revised edn 2012.

Williams, Meg Harris, *The Aesthetic Development: The Poetic Spirit of Psychoanalysis: Essays on Bion, Melzer, Keats*, London: Karnac Books Ltd., 2010.

Wilson, Eric G., *How to Make a Soul: The Wisdom of John Keats*, Evanston: Northwestern University Press, 2016, 18.

Wolfson Susan J. (ed.), *The Cambridge Companion to Keats*, Cambridge: Cambridge University Press, 2001.

Wolfson, Susan, 'Keats's "Gordian Complication" of Women', in Walter H. Evert and Jack W. Rhodes (eds) ,*Approaches to Teaching Keats's Poetry*, New York: *The Modern Language Association of America*, 1991, 77–85.

Wolfson, Susan, "Feminizing Keats", in Hermione de Almeida (ed.), *Critical Essays on John Keats*, Boston: G. K. Hall, 1990, 317–56.

Young, Edward, *The Complaint and the Consolation; Or, Night Thoughts*, London: R. Noble, 1797, 5.

'Z', 'The Cockney School of Poetry, no. iv', *Blackwood's Edinburgh Magazine*, 3 (1818) 519–24, 519.

Ziegenhagen, Timothy, 'Keats, Professional Medicine, and the Two Hyperions', *Literature and Medicine*, 21 (2002), 281–305.

Index